P9-DTS-686

NCLEX-RN
VOCABULARY & MEDICATIONS FLASHCARDS

Premium Edition

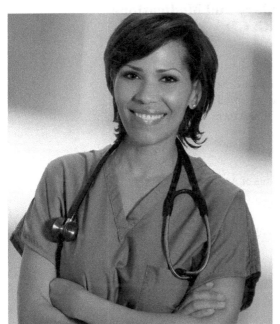

Michael Adams, Ph.D.
Jeanine Brice, RN, BSN

 Research & Education Association
Visit our website at: www.rea.com

Research & Education Association
61 Ethel Road West
Piscataway, New Jersey 08854
E-mail: info@rea.com

NCLEX-RN Vocabulary and Medications Flashcard Book with CD

Published 2012

Copyright © 2011 by Research & Education Association, Inc. All rights reserved. No part of this book may be reproduced in any form without permission of the publisher.

Printed in the United States of America

ISBN-13: 978-0-7386-0905-8
ISBN-10: 0-7386-0905-6

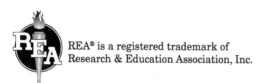

REA® is a registered trademark of Research & Education Association, Inc.

From the Authors

The National Council Licensure Examination (NCLEX) is the culmination of the total knowledge, skills, and abilities learned in nursing school. It is recognized as a significant milestone in an individual's entry into professional nursing practice.

One of the most frequent questions from students is how best to prepare for (and pass) the NCLEX-RN® examination. From your first weeks in nursing school, your instructors began preparing you for this examination. Throughout your classes, important information was stressed: This is information that you will use to practice nursing safely, effectively, and compassionately.

Now, the rest is up to you. Reviewing this extensive body of knowledge is a long process, and it is never easy. To assist you in focusing on important aspects of your nursing education, we have created a listing of over 400 key vocabulary terms and medications that are most likely to appear on the NCLEX-RN® exam. Term and medication information is presented in a handy flashcard format in order to help you (and your study group) memorize and understand each term with ease. Although questions may vary on each examination, these terms and medications are fundamental to nursing practice. They were created to help you focus on core concepts that are encountered on the exam.

The medications selected for inclusion are those most frequently prescribed in the United States. Information is supplied in a concise format, outlining the drug name (generic and brand), pronunciation, drug classification, side effects, and nursing implications and precautions.

The key vocabulary terms were selected from the NCSBN 2010 RN Test Plan and are classified according to the steps of the nursing process. Terms related to illness were identified as some of the most common diseases/disorders found in the United States. Along with the key term is a pronunciation, the definition, and a sentence that provides an example of its use in nursing practice.

As authors, it is our hope that these flashcards will help to increase your score and accomplish a major goal in your future career. Best wishes for much success!

Michael Adams, Ph.D.

Jeanine Brice, RN, BSN

About the Authors

Dr. Michael Adams has authored three textbooks in pharmacology: *Core Concepts in Pharmacology* by Holland & Adams; *Pharmacology: a Pathophysiology Approach* by Adams, Holland, and Urban; and *Pharmacology: Connections to Nursing Practice* by Adams and Koch. Dr. Adams has an M.S. degree in Pharmacology from Michigan State University and a Ph.D. in Curriculum and Instruction from the University of South Florida. He is currently Professor of Biological Sciences at Pasco-Hernando Community College in New Port Richey, Florida.

Jeanine Brice is currently an Associate Professor and Coordinator of Technical Health programs at Pasco-Hernando Community College in New Port Richey, Florida. She has been a registered nurse for over 23 years and has been involved in nursing education for the last 20 years, providing didactic and clinical instruction to nursing students. Her nursing and clinical education experiences include those in medical, surgical, long-term care, pediatrics, and obstetrics units. Ms. Brice has an ADN from Charles County Community College (College of Southern Maryland), a B.S. from the University of Maryland, and an M.S. in Nursing Education/Community Health from Bowie State University.

Table of Contents

About Research & Education Association

Founded in 1959, Research & Education Association (REA) is dedicated to publishing the finest and most effective educational materials—including software, study guides, and test preps—for students in elementary school, middle school, high school, college, graduate school, and beyond.

Today, REA's wide-ranging catalog is a leading resource for teachers, students, and professionals.

We invite you to visit us at *www.rea.com* to find out how "REA is making the world smarter."

Acknowledgments

In addition to our authors, we would like to thank Pam Weston, Publisher, for setting the quality standards for production integrity and managing the publication to completion; Larry B. Kling, Vice President, Editorial, for his overall direction; Michael Reynolds, Managing Editor, for project management; Christine Saul, Senior Graphic Artist, for designing our cover; and S4Carlisle for typesetting this edition.

Absorption
(ab-SORBT-shun)

Nursing Process Category: All

Acquired Immune Deficiency Syndrome (AIDS)
(ah-KWIRED ih-MUNE dih-FISH-en-see SIN-drome)

Nursing Process Category: Assessment

Activities of Daily Living (ADLs)
(ahk-TIV-ih-tees of DAY-lee LIV-ing)

Nursing Process Category: Assessment

Absorption is the first step in the movement of a drug through the body, the process by which a drug passes into the client's bloodstream.

*The nurse must ensure that the correct form of the drug is given by the route intended in order for **absorption** to occur.*

AIDS is an immune disorder caused by infection by the human immunodeficiency virus (HIV), and is characterized by increased susceptibility to opportunistic infections and rare cancers.

*The nurse is aware, and educates clients, that symptoms of **acquired immune deficiency syndrome (AIDS)** may appear anytime from several months to several years after acquiring HIV.*

ADLs are activities typically performed in the course of a normal day. Such activities include eating, bathing, toileting, and dressing.

*The ability to perform **activities of daily living (ADLs)** may be inhibited by illness or injury.*

Actual Problem
(AK-choo-al PROB-lum)

Nursing Process Category: Nursing Diagnosis

Acute Illness
(ah-CUTE ILL-ness)

Nursing Process Category: Assessment

Adaptation
(ah-DAPT-ay-shun)

Nursing Process Category: All

An actual problem is a problem that exists now; it is present and current.

*The client is currently experiencing an **actual problem**. He is having pain in his foot, which is affecting his gait.*

An acute illness is characterized by intense symptoms of relatively short duration.

*During assessment, the nurse assesses the client's symptoms to determine whether the illness is **acute** or chronic.*

Adaptation is coping behavior that provides the ability to handle the demands of a changing environment, situation, or illness.

*The nurse assesses the client's **adaptation** abilities when developing teaching strategies.*

Addiction
(ad-ICT-shun)

Nursing Process Category: Assessment

Adolescence
(ah-doll-ESS-ense)

Nursing Process Category: Assessment

Adult
(ad-ULT)

Nursing Process Category: Assessment

Addiction is a compulsive and maladaptive dependence on a substance despite negative physical, social, emotional, and economic implications. Substances can include alcohol, cocaine, opiates, or tobacco; also may be a behavior such as gambling.

*The nurse learns that the client continues to use alcohol despite physical harm to the client and a negative impact on the client's family life, and determines that the client may have an **addiction** to alcohol.*

Adolescence is the period of development spanning the ages of 12 to 18 years, characterized by becoming physically and psychologically mature, acquiring a personal identity, and preparing for adulthood and associated responsibilities.

*The nurse understands that the principal risks during **adolescence** are due to the consequences of risky behavior, such as injury related to accidents, drug experimentation, and teen pregnancy.*

Adult (or adulthood) is a period of development spanning from age 20 to 65 years, encompassing the young adult period (20 to 40 years of age) and middle age (40 to 65 years of age).

*The nurses use knowledge of growth and development when caring for **adult** clients to determine safety needs, approach to care and client teaching, and health promotion needs.*

Advance Directive
(ad-VANCE dih-REK-tiv)

Nursing Process Category: Implementation

Adverse Drug Reaction/Adverse Drug Event (ADE)
(AD-verse drug ree-AK-shun)

Nursing Process Category: Assessment

Advocate
(AD-vo-kat)

Nursing Process Category: Implementation

An advance directive is a legal document (or documents) that allows persons to specify specific aspects of care should they become unable to communicate their preferences.

*All health care facilities that receive Medicare and Medicaid reimbursement must recognize **advance directives,** according to the Patient Self-Determination Act of 1991.*

An adverse drug reaction (or adverse drug event) is an unwanted response to a pharmaceutical drug.

*Health professionals are encouraged to report all **adverse drug reactions**/events related to drugs or medical devices to the manufacturer and the Food and Drug Administration (FDA). Monitoring for such **adverse drug reactions** is a vital part of the nursing role.*

An advocate is a person who speaks or writes in support of another person. This is a major role of the nurse.

*The nurse is an **advocate** for the client, ensuring that the rights of the client are accommodated.*

Aging
(AGE-ing)

Nursing Process Category: Assessment

Alzheimer's Disease
(ALLS-hime-ers diz-EEZ)

Nursing Process Category: Assessment

Anemia
(ah-NEEM-ee-ah)

Nursing Process Category: Assessment

Aging is the process of growing older and maturing, and sometimes refers to the physical changes that occur with time rather than from injury or disease.

Aging is associated with a number of physical changes, including changes to the integumentary, neuromuscular, sensory/perceptual, pulmonary, cardiovascular, gastrointestinal, and genitourinary systems.

Alzheimer's disease is the most common form of dementia, which is a progressive loss of cognitive function.

*The at-home caregivers of clients with **Alzheimer's disease** may experience physical and emotional exhaustion while they render the sometimes continuous care needed for the person with Alzheimer's disease.*

Anemia is a reduction in the number of circulating red blood cells, affecting tissue oxygenation.

*Signs of **anemia** may include chronic fatigue, pallor, shortness of breath, and hypotension.*

Anxiety Disorder
(anks-EYE-ih-tee diss-OAR-der)

Nursing Process Category: Assessment

Apgar Score
(AHP-garr skore)

Nursing Process Category: Assessment

Appendicitis
(app-END-iss-EYE-tiss)

Nursing Process Category: Assessment

Anxiety disorder is a common reaction to stress characterized by mental uneasiness, apprehension, or dread related to an impending or anticipated, yet unidentified, threat to self or significant relationships.

*The nurse can help clients with an **anxiety disorder** to identify situations that precipitate anxiety and identify signs of anxiety.*

The Apgar score is a system used to assess newborn infants within 60 seconds after birth, and is repeated 5 minutes later. It provides a numeric indicator of the infant's physiologic capacities to adapt to extrauterine life.

*The nurse recognizes that the maximum **Apgar score** is 10, and a score under 7 indicates that the infant is having difficulty.*

Appendicitis is an inflammation of the vermiform appendix, which often requires surgery to remove the appendix.

*The nurse must assess for **appendicitis** carefully, because many other conditions can cause abdominal pain.*

Arrhythmia
(ay-RITH-mia)

Nursing Process Category: Assessment

Assessment
(uh-SES-ment)

Nursing Process Category: Assessment

Asthma
(ASTH-mah)

Nursing Process Category: Assessment

An arrhythmia is a pulse with an irregular rhythm. Also called *dysrhythmia*.

*The nurse should assess the apical pulse when an **arrhythmia** is detected.*

Assessment is the first step in the nursing process in which the nurse gathers complete, holistic client information in order to identify actual and/or potential problems, then plan and implement care.

*Before providing care, the nurse must complete a client **assessment** in order to meet the client's needs.*

Asthma involves episodic inflammation and narrowing of the airways in response to a variety of stimuli.

*The nurse is responsible for teaching proper use of **asthma** medications to clients.*

Auscultation
(AH-skull-TAY-shun)

Auscultate
(AH-skull-tate)

Nursing Process Category: Assessment

Basic Human Needs
(BAY-sik HUE-man NEEDZ)

Nursing Process Category: All

Benign Prostatic Hypertrophy (BPH)
(bee-NINE prost-AT-tik HY-purr-troh-phee)

Nursing Process Category: Assessment

Auscultation is a method of listening to the sounds of the body (lungs, heart, and intestines) during a physical examination usually done using a stethoscope. Nurses routinely listen to evaluate the frequency, intensity, duration, number, and quality of sounds.

*The correct method of **auscultation** of breath sounds is to listen to the chest with a stethoscope, comparing one side to the other side.*

Basic human needs include elements required for survival and normal mental and physical health. These factors include food, water, shelter, and protection from the environment. Maslow's Hierarchy of Needs theory categorizes human needs according to the most important needs for survival. Basic human needs on the hierarchy scale are referred to as "physiologic."

*Nurses need to realize that their clients' most **basic human needs** must be addressed first before higher level needs can be met.*

Benign prostatic hypertrophy is an enlargement of the prostate gland, and is the most common benign (nonmalignant) neoplasm in aging men.

*In **benign prostatic hypertrophy (BPH)**, prostate nodules enlarge around the urethra, which causes the common symptoms of urinary frequency, difficulty starting or stopping the urine stream, or urinary urgency.*

Birth
(burrth)

Nursing Process Category: All

Body Mechanics
(BOD-ee mek-AN-iks)

Nursing Process Category: Implementation

Bowel Training
(BOW-ull TREY-ning)

Nursing Process Category: Implementation

Birth is the normal physiologic process of passing a child from the uterus, or the act of being born.

*The four stages of labor and vaginal **birth** include the first stage, which is divided into the latent, active, and transition phases; the second stage, which begins when the cervix is completely dilated (10 cm); the third stage, which is from the birth of the infant to the completed delivery of the placenta; and the fourth stage, which lasts 1 to 4 hours after the expulsion of the placenta.*

Body mechanics describe the safe use of the body to move objects and perform the activities of daily living.

*Although careful attention to **body mechanics** is important for nurses, the nursing field still ranks sixth in the most at-risk occupations for back injuries.*

Bowel training is a method of establishing regular bowel evacuation by reflex conditioning. This technique is used for the treatment of fecal incontinence, impaction, chronic diarrhea, and autonomic hyperreflexia.

*After a spinal cord injury, a male client suffered quadriplegia. As a result of the client's paralysis, he also developed autonomic hyperreflexia, a neurologic disorder that stimulates the intestinal tract. To assist with this condition, the nurse uses a **bowel training** program.*

Breast Cancer
(BREAST kan-serr)

Nursing Process Category: Assessment

Bulimia
(bull-EEM-ia)

Nursing Process Category: Assessment

Case Management
(KASE MAN-aj-ment)

Nursing Process Category: All

Breast cancer is a malignant neoplasm of the breast tissue.

*The risk of **breast cancer** increases with age, and is the most frequently diagnosed cancer in women. In the United States, the lifetime risk of developing **breast cancer** for women is 1 in 8.*

Bulimia is an eating disorder characterized by bingeing on food (secretly consuming large quantities of food), then purging.

*The treatment of eating disorders such as **bulimia** is best accomplished through a team approach, including nutritional, medical, and psychiatric practitioners familiar with eating disorders.*

Case management is a range of models that integrate health care services for individuals or groups and involves interdisciplinary teams of practitioners.

*In **case management**, the manager may be a nurse, social worker, or other appropriate professional.*

Cerebrovascular Accident (CVA)
(seh-REE-bro-vask-yoo-lar AX-ih-dent)

Nursing Process Category: Assessment

Cervical Cancer
(SIR-vik-al KAN-sir)

Nursing Process Category: Assessment

Child Abuse
(CHEYE-ild AB-use)

Nursing Process Category: Assessment

A cerebrovascular accident is a loss of blood flow to an area of the brain that causes a sudden loss of neurologic function; also called *stroke*.

*Common signs of **cerebrovascular accident (CVA)** include speech problems, paralysis or weakness on one side of the body, vision problems, and/or memory loss.*

Cervical cancer is a malignant lesion of the cervix.

*The Pap test is used to assess abnormal cells on the cervix, and is a screening tool for **cervical cancer.***

Child abuse is the physical, sexual, or emotional mistreatment (including neglect) of a child.

*Nurses are legally responsible for reporting a case of suspected **child abuse.***

Cholecystitis
(KOLE-ee-siss-tye-tis)

Nursing Process Category: Assessment

Chronic Illness
(KRON-ik ILL-ness)

Nursing Process Category: Assessment

Clear Liquid Diet
(KLEER LIK-wid DYE-it)

Nursing Process Category: Implementation

Cholecystitis is the inflammátion of the gallbladder.

*The most common symptom of **cholecystitis** is pain in the upper right quadrant of the abdomen shortly after eating.*

A chronic illness is one that lasts for an extended period, usually for 6 months or longer, and can often last for the person's life.

*Nurses care for clients with **chronic illness** of all ages and in all types of settings, including homes, nursing homes, hospitals, and others.*

A clear liquid diet is a type of short term, special diet that is limited to water, tea, coffee, clear broths, ginger ale, juices, and plain gelatin.

*The main goal of a **clear liquid diet** is to prevent dehydration and minimize stimulation of the gastrointestinal tract.*

Client (Patient) Education
(KLY-ent) (ed-u-KAY-shun)

Nursing Process Category: Implementation

Client Rights
(KLEYE-ent RITES)

Nursing Process Category: All

Code of Ethics
(KODE of ETH-iks)

Nursing Process Category: All

Client education (or patient education) is a major nursing function. It involves providing information to a client in a teaching-learning environment where the nurse and client work together to better the client's health status.

*The client, age 16, has just been diagnosed with diabetes. The nurse assigned for the care of the client is responsible for establishing a **client education** session with her to make sure she understands her newly diagnosed condition.*

Client rights (also called patient rights) include the right for clients to make choices and decisions relating to their health care, and to expect a nurse-client relationship based on respect, trust, collaboration, and consideration of their thoughts and feelings. Additional rights specific to clients' health insurance plans were mandated in a piece of legislation passed in 2004 (the Patients' Bill of Rights Act of 2004).

*The goal of the nurse as client advocate is to protect **client rights.***

A code of ethics is a formal statement of ideals and values.

*The nursing **code of ethics** serves as a standard and guideline for nurses' professional actions and informs the public of its commitment to their ideals and values.*

Collaborate
(kuh-LAB-uh-rate)

Nursing Process Category: Planning

Comfort Measures
(KUM-fert MEH-zures)

Nursing Process Category: Implementation

Communication
(ko-muhn-ih-KAY-shun)

Nursing Process Category: All

To collaborate is to work with one with another; to cooperate.

*The nurse and client **collaborate** with one another to develop a plan of care for the client.*

To comfort is to soothe, console, or reassure. The nurse demonstrates a caring attitude and implements measures to helps to reduce client anxiety and assist in relaxation. Measures are individualized to the client and situation.

*Listening, use of massage, facilitated breathing, and use of medications are several ways the nurse can provide **comfort measures** for the client.*

Communication is the exchange of thoughts or information by speech, writing, and/or signs. Many factors, such as age, education, culture, relationships, and environment can influence the effectiveness of communication.

*Nurses realize that in order for **communication** to be effective, they need to use language that the client can understand.*

Confidentiality
(KON-fid-ent-ee-al-ity)

Nursing Process Category: All

Conflict(s)
(KON-flikt)

Nursing Process Category: Planning

Conflict Resolution
(KON-flikt rez-oh-LU-shun)

Nursing Process Category: Implementation

Confidentiality is the protection of information that one wishes to keep private, such as health information.

*A nurse demonstrates **confidentiality** by not giving information about clients over the phone unless the client has signed a form giving permission for private health information to be shared with that exact person.*

A conflict is an incompatibility or disagreement over an idea, desire, event, or activity with another. Conflict is not always an indication of a negative situation, but at times can allow for the formation of creative ideas and solutions.

*The client has been diagnosed with a terminal disease. She has been given several treatment alternatives and is having a **conflict** regarding which treatment to choose.*

Conflict resolution is the process of settling an incompatibility or disagreement. Several approaches are used and all involve critical-thinking abilities. Some approaches include accommodation, avoidance, collaboration, competition, and compromise.

*A nurse manager assigns two nurses to work together to solve a specific problem on their hospital unit. The nurses choose the **conflict resolution** approach of collaboration to solve the problem.*

Continuity of Care
(KON-tin-ooh-it-ee of KARE)

Nursing Process Category: Implementation and Evaluation

Contraception
(KON-trah-cep-shun)

Nursing Process Category: Implementation

Contraindication
(KON-trah-in-dih-kay-shun)

Nursing Process Category: Planning & Implementation

Continuity of care is the coordination of health care for clients who move from one health setting to another, and between and among health care practitioners.

*When clients are admitted to any health care setting, the nurse provides **continuity of care** by initiating discharge planning, involving the client and family in the planning process, and collaborating with other health care practitioners.*

Contraception is the prevention of unwanted pregnancy.

*The nurse discusses with the woman factors that the woman should consider in choosing a method of **contraception.***

A contraindication is any symptom, preexisting condition, or circumstance that makes treatment with a drug or medical device unsafe.

*When administering medications, the nurse must be aware of any **contraindication** to the client taking that drug before administering the drug.*

Coping Mechanism
(KOH-ping MECK-an-izm)

Nursing Process Category: Evaluation

Crisis Intervention
(CRY-sis IN-terr-vent-shun)

Nursing Process Category: Implementation

Culture
(KUL-cher)

Nursing Process Category: Planning

A coping mechanism is a natural or learned way, either through action or relieving emotional distress, of responding to the environment, problem, or situation. Also called a *coping strategy*. Can be long term or short term.

The client states to the nurse that he does not talk with his family or friends about his recent cancer diagnosis. The nurse recognizes that the client is using an avoidance **coping mechanism** *to manage the stress of his situation.*

A crisis intervention is a short term process of helping clients to resolve a crisis and restore the client's precrisis level of functioning.

During a **crisis intervention,** *the nurse uses steps that mirror the steps of the nursing process.*

Culture relates to the behaviors and beliefs characteristic of a particular social, ethnic, or age group.

It is important that the nurse be aware of the differences in **culture** *so the client's rights and needs are fulfilled.*

Cushing's Syndrome
(KUSH-ings SIN-drome)

Nursing Process Category: Assessment

Cystic Fibrosis (CF)
(SISS-tik FYE-broh-siss)

Nursing Process Category: Assessment

Deep Vein Thrombosis (DVT)
(DEEP VAYN THROM-bow-siss)

Nursing Process Category: Assessment

Cushing's syndrome results from prolonged exposure to glucocorticoids, either from those naturally excreted by the adrenal glands or from glucocorticoid administration.

*During the physical assessment of the client with **Cushing's syndrome,** the nurse may note excessive fat in the face, upper back, and trunk; abdominal skin may have striae (purplish lines); hypertension may be present; and women may have excessive hair growth on the face and extremities.*

Cystic fibrosis is a disease that causes chronic obstructive pulmonary disease, frequent lung infections, deficient pancreatic enzymes, and abnormally high electrolytes in the client's sweat.

*The nurse teaches the client with **cystic fibrosis,** as well as the client's family, how to perform pulmonary chest physiotherapy and postural drainage that are necessary to mobilize secretions.*

A deep vein thrombosis is a stationary clot that forms in the veins of the leg.

*The nurse may implement interventions to prevent **deep vein thrombosis (DVT)** such as early ambulation, pneumatic compression stockings, or anticoagulant medications.*

Delegation
(del-ih-GAY-shun)
Delegate
(del-ih-GATE)

Nursing Process Category: Implementation

Depression
(dee-PRESH-un)

Nursing Process Category: Assessment

Dermatitis
(der-mah-TITE-iss)

Nursing Process Category: Assessment

Delegation (to delegate) is to give responsibilities (powers and functions) to another person.

*As part of the health care team, the nurse frequently **delegates** some client care responsibilities to a nursing assistant.*

Depression is a mood disorder characterized by lack of energy, depressed mood, sleep disturbances, and feelings of hopelessness, guilt, and despair.

*The nurse should perform a detailed assessment to determine whether the client is experiencing **depression,** because certain drugs, and other medical and neurologic disorders may mimic the symptoms of depression.*

Dermatitis is an inflammation of the skin that produces an itchy, red rash.

*Antihistamine medications are often prescribed for **dermatitis,** and the nurse should advise clients that these medications can cause drowsiness and the client should avoid operating any type of equipment (including driving).*

Developmental Stages
(dee-vell-ahp-MENT-all STAY-gez)

Nursing Process Category: All

Diabetes Mellitus (DM)
(die-ah-BEET-eez mell-EYE-tiss)

Nursing Process Category: Assessment

Diverticular Disease
(die-verr-TIK-u-lar dis-EEZ)

Nursing Process Category: Assessment

There are several theories regarding the various stages of human growth and development, but the most well-known are Erikson's eight stages of development, which range from infancy and early childhood to adulthood and maturity. In Erikson's theory, each developmental stage signals a task that must be accomplished, and the nurse assesses indicators of positive and negative resolution of each stage.

*Identifying clients' **developmental stages** help nurses to identify predictable patterns of characteristics and nursing implications to develop appropriate plans of care.*

Diabetes mellitus is a chronic metabolic disease characterized by hyperglycemia, and is comprised of two types: type 1 DM is caused by a lack of secretion of insulin by the pancreas; type 2 DM is caused by insufficient secretion of insulin by the pancreas and insulin receptors that lack sensitivity to insulin.

*The 55-year-old male client has recently been diagnosed with **diabetes mellitus (DM)**. The nurse recognizes that this diagnosis increases the client's risk of coronary heart disease, myocardial infarction, and peripheral vascular disease.*

Diverticular disease is characterized by development of small sacs (or pockets) in the colon wall known as diverticula, and is comprised of three conditions that include diverticulitis (inflammation and infection of the diverticula), bleeding of the diverticula, and diverticulosis (numerous diverticula).

*The nurse teaches the client with **diverticular disease** ways to change diet and lifestyle habits in order to control the condition.*

Documentation
(dok-u-men-TAY-shun)
Document(s)
(DOK-u-ment)

Nursing Process Category: Implementation

Drip Rate
(DRIP RAYT)

Nursing Process Category: Implementation

Drug Action
(DRUG ACK-shun)

Nursing Process Category: All

To document is to record client information and nursing care in order to substantiate that certain information and care was provided. It also acts as a document that is used to make health care decisions and provide continuity of care. Documentation is usually done via computer program or hard copy (paper) forms.

After conducting a client assessment, the nurse immediately **documents** *the findings on the hospital's computer documentation system.*

In intravenous infusions, the drip rate (also called the drip factor or drop factor) is the number of drops delivered per milliliter of solution.

The **drip rate** *is generally printed on the package of the intravenous infusion set.*

Drug action is how a drug functions in various body systems. It is sometimes called *mechanism of action*, which is the means by which a drug exerts its effect on the cells or tissues.

Understanding **drug action** *helps the nurse to ensure safe drug administration.*

Drug Dependence
(DRUG dee-PEND-ense)

Nursing Process Category: Assessment

Drug Tolerance
(DRUG TALL-err-anse)

Nursing Process Category: Assessment

Electrolyte
(ee-LEK-troh-light)

Nursing Process Category: Implementation

Drug dependence is a strong physiologic or psychologic need for a drug.

*The nurse should discern between the two types of **drug dependence**: physical dependence, which produces sometimes severe physical symptoms upon withdrawal of the drug; and psychologic dependence, which produces no signs of physical discomfort upon withdrawal, but the user continues to feel an overwhelming desire for the drug.*

Drug tolerance is the process of adapting to a drug over time, which results in a need to increase dosages of the drug to achieve the same effect.

*The nurse should discern between **drug tolerance**, dependence, and addiction—especially in pain management—for clients.*

An electrolyte is a charged particle that is part of the body's fluid, and is capable of conducting electricity. The balance of electrolytes—most notably sodium, potassium, chloride, and bicarbonate—is essential to the normal functioning of the body.

*The nurse understands that infants and children, and older adults, are at high risk for **electrolyte** imbalances.*

Emphysema
(EM-phiz-EE-mah)

Nursing Process Category: Assessment

Endometriosis
(EN-doh-meet-tree-OH-siss)

Nursing Process Category: Assessment

Epidural
(EH-pee-DOO-rall)

Nursing Process Category: Implementation

Emphysema is a chronic obstructive pulmonary disease in which the alveoli of the lungs are distended, causing difficulty in exhaling air with chronically elevated carbon dioxide levels.

*In clients with **emphysema**, decreased oxygen concentrations due to chronically elevated carbon dioxide levels are the main stimuli for respiration.*

Endometriosis is a condition in which endometrial tissue grows outside the uterine cavity, most commonly in the pelvic cavity. This extrauterine tissue responds to the hormonal changes of the menstrual cycle and bleeds in a cyclic fashion, which can result in symptoms such as pain and infertility.

*Treatment for **endometriosis** may be pharmacologic or surgical, or a combination of the two.*

Epidural is a route of parenteral medication administration near the base of the spine, most commonly used for administering an anesthetic for pain management. It is most often administered for pain relief during the first and second stages of labor, but is also used for pain relief in other situations.

*After **epidural** anesthesia is administered during labor, the nurse assesses the woman's level of pain relief.*

Epilepsy
(EH-pill-EP-see)

Nursing Process Category: Assessment

Ethical
(ETH-ih-kal)

Nursing Process Category: Implementation

Evaluation
(EE-val-you-AY-shun)
Evaluate
(ee-VAL-you-ate)

Nursing Process Category: Evaluation

Epilepsy is a disease that involves chronic seizure activity (that is, repetitive, abnormal discharge of electrical activity within the brain).

*Medications used to treat **epilepsy** must be given continuously and on time throughout the client's life to maintain therapeutic blood levels.*

Being ethical is acting in accordance with a set of standards (ethics) of conduct. Nursing organizations have established a code of conduct that provides ethical guidelines for nursing practice.

*It is not **ethical** for nurses to provide client information without the consent of the client or his/her legal representative.*

Evaluation is the fifth step of the nursing process, and is the systematic process for determining whether a client goal has been achieved or a nursing intervention has been effective.

*The nursing process step of **evaluation** is conducted by the nurse when the nurse asks the client, "Was your pain relieved by the medication you received?"*

Exercise
(EKS-err-size)

Nursing Process Category: Implementation

Family-Centered Nursing
(FAM-ih-lee SENT-urd NUR-sing)

Nursing Process Category: All

Fluid Balance
(FLOO-id BAL-anse)

Nursing Process Category: Implementation

Exercise is physical activity done with the goal of improving one or more components of physical fitness.

*The nurse must assess each client for his or her tolerance to activity when planning an individualized **exercise** prescription.*

Family-centered nursing considers the health of the family as a unit, in addition to the health of individual family members. The nurse can better plan a client's care with an understanding of family dynamics.

*A key component of **family-centered nursing** is the family assessment, which determines the family structure, roles and functions, physical health status, interaction patterns, values, and coping resources.*

The goal of fluid balance is to regulate the amount of liquid in the body, striving for equilibrium rather than too little fluid (fluid deficit) or too much fluid (fluid overload).

*The nurse monitors a client's **fluid balance** by measuring intake and output (I&O) as well as by measuring day-to-day variations in body weight.*

Fluid Retention

(FLOO-id ree-TEN-shun)

Nursing Process Category: Assessment

Fluid Therapy

(FLOO-id THER-uh-pee)

Nursing Process Category: Implementation

General Anesthesia

(JEN-ral AN-ess-THEES-ee-ah)

Nursing Process Category: Implementation

Fluid retention (or *fluid volume excess*) is a result of the body's failure to eliminate fluid due to renal, cardiac, and/or metabolic disease.

*The nurse may counsel the client with **fluid retention** in dietary changes such as a low-sodium diet.*

Fluid therapy is the regulation of water balance in clients with gastrointestinal, renal, cardiac or metabolic impairment by measuring fluid intake (oral liquids, IV fluids) against losses (urination, vomiting). If losses exceed intake, fluid replacement will be needed.

***Fluid therapy** via an intravenous (IV) line and delivery of 0.9% NS (normal saline) is initiated on the client because she had been vomiting for approximately 24 hours and became dehydrated.*

Anesthesia is the partial or complete loss of sensation, and general anesthesia produces a *complete* loss of sensation (unconsciousness). It is also referred to as a *medically controlled coma.*

*When a client emerges from **general anesthesia,** the nurse protects the client's airway and monitors the client's vital signs. The nurse then evaluates level of consciousness (LOC), reflex status, motor activity, and orients the client to person, place, and time as necessary.*

Goal(s)
(gohl)

Nursing Process Category: Planning

Grief
(GREEF)

Nursing Process Category: Assessment

Hazardous Materials ("HAZ MAT")
(HAZ-ar-duss mah-TEAR-ee-alls)

Nursing Process Category: Assessment

Goals are desired results, or the achievement toward which effort is directed. In nursing, client goals are described in terms of a broad statement of observable client responses and effort usually includes nursing interventions.

*When developing the nursing care plan, the nurse and client establish the following **goal:** the client will be free from pain.*

Grief is emotional suffering that often follows the loss of a loved person or thing.

*It is important for the nurse to assist clients experiencing **grief** to work through their feelings because prolonged grief may have potentially devastating effects on health.*

Hazardous materials in health care refer to any tissue or substance that could endanger health, including lead, asbestos, needles, body fluids, surgical sponges, human waste, some pharmaceuticals (such as chemotherapeutic agents), and radioisotopes.

*In order to prevent endangering public health, **hazardous materials** must be properly labeled, handled, and disposed of.*

Head Injury
(HED IN-jur-ee)

Nursing Process Category: Assessment

Health Screening
(HELTH SCREE-ning)

Nursing Process Category: Assessment

Heart Failure
(HART FAIL-yoor)

Nursing Process Category: Assessment

Head injury is any trauma to the head that may cause soft tissue damage or internal injury to the brain, and often occurs as a result of motor vehicle crashes, falls, and sports. It is also called *traumatic brain injury.*

Head injury *is one of the most common causes of death and disability in the United States.*

A health screening (also known as a *health risk appraisal*) is a test to assess specific areas of physical growth, development, and health status. Different health screenings are done at each age/ developmental stage.

*People over the age of 50 are recommended to have the **health screening** test for colon cancer, a colonoscopy.*

Heart failure is the inability of the heart to pump sufficient blood to meet the body's needs. Symptoms include shortness of breath, cold and pale extremities, and a persistent, dry cough due to fluid congestion in the lungs.

*In African Americans, symptoms of **heart failure** often occur earlier, which is possibly due to the higher rate of uncontrolled high blood pressure (hypertension).*

Herpes
(HER-peez)

Nursing Process Category: Assessment

Holistic Care
(hol-IS-tik KARE)

Nursing Process Category: All

Hormone Replacement Therapy (HRT)
(HOR-mone ree-PLACE-ment THAIR-ah-pee)

Nursing Process Category: Implementation

Herpes is a skin eruption caused by one of the two families of *herpesvirus*, herpes simplex or herpes zoster.

*The goal of standard precautions in care of the client with **herpes** is to prevent spread of the virus.*

Holistic care focuses on the whole person, integrating prevention, treatment, and management of illness or disease and the preservation, maintenance, or restoration of mental, physical, and spiritual health using both conventional and alternative therapies.

*Using a **holistic care** approach for his or her client, the nurse addresses the needs of the whole person rather than just a specific area.*

Used to treat symptoms of menopause, hormone replacement therapy involves the administration of estrogen and progestin combination medications.

*The nurse recognizes that one of the risks with **hormone replacement therapy (HRT)** is increased risk of heart disease, pulmonary embolism, stroke, and breast and endometrial cancers.*

Human Immunodeficiency Virus (HIV)
(HYOO-man ih-MUNE-oh-dih-FISH-en-see VY-russ)

Nursing Process Category: Assessment

Human Papilloma Virus (HPV)
(HYOO-man PAP-ill-OH-mah VY-russ)

Nursing Process Category: Assessment

Hygiene Needs
(HIGH-jeen NEEDZ)

Nursing Process Category: Implementation

Human immunodeficiency virus is a retrovirus that causes acquired immune deficiency syndrome (AIDS), leading to a loss of immune function and subsequent development of opportunistic infections.

*A postexposure protocol (PEP) is implemented after occupational exposure to **human immunodeficiency virus (HIV),** which involves drug treatment and ongoing HIV antibody tests.*

Human papilloma virus is a common sexually transmitted disease, and a number of subtypes have been shown to contribute to cancers of the anus, cervix, penis, and vulva.

*The Gardasil vaccine has been proven to be effective in preventing two of the strains of **human papilloma virus (HPV)** responsible for a large percentage of cervical cancer cases.*

Hygiene is the science of health and sanitation, and a client's hygiene needs include tasks such as regular bathing, nail trimming, and oral cleansing.

Hygiene needs *become even more important for immobile clients, or those with cognitive disabilities such as dementia.*

Hypertension
(HIGH-perr-TEN-shun)

Nursing Process Category: Assessment

Hyperthyroidism
(HIGH-perr-THIGH-roid-izm)

Nursing Process Category: Assessment

Hypothyroidism
(HIGH-poh-THIGH-roid-izm)

Nursing Process Category: Assessment

Hypertension (also known as high blood pressure) is a condition in which blood pressure is abnormally high. In adults, hypertension is diagnosed with blood pressure (BP) readings higher than 140 mmHg systolic or 90 mmHg diastolic after three separate readings that are recorded several weeks apart.

Hypertension is sometimes called a "silent" disease because many clients are symptom free until complications arise, which can occur decades after the hypertension first begins.

Hyperthyroidism is a disease characterized by abnormally high levels of thyroid hormone in the body. The most common cause is Graves' disease.

Treatments for hyperthyroidism include destruction of the thyroid gland with radioactive iodine, surgical removal of the thyroid, or antithyroid drugs.

Hypothyroidism is a condition that results from inadequate levels of thyroid hormone in the body.

Treatment for hypothyroidism typically is lifelong administration of thyroid hormone.

Immobility
(IH-moh-BILL-ih-tee)

Nursing Process Category: Assessment

Immunization
(IM-yoon-iz-AY-shun)

Nursing Process Category: Implementation

Implementation
(IM-pluh-men-TAY-shun)
Implement
(IM-pluh-ment)

Nursing Process Category: Implementation

Immobility or inactivity is usually due to a sedentary lifestyle, illness, or injury. The duration of inactivity, the client's sense of awareness, and the client's general health condition can increase the risk for long term complications.

Immobility affects all body systems; therefore, the nurse needs to be alert and attentive to any changes and provide for the needs of their clients. Example: Turning an immobile client every 2 hours helps to prevent pressure ulcers.

Immunization (sometimes also called *vaccination*) is the process of administering a substance via the oral or parenteral route that confers to the recipient resistance to that substance.

The Centers for Disease Control (CDC) publishes a recommended schedule of immunization for children, adolescents, and adults.

Implementation is the fourth step in the nursing process. It includes the actual providing of care and documentation of nursing actions, as indicated in the nursing care plan.

Implementation occurs when the nurse initiates and completes a nursing action such as the administration of medication.

Impotence
(IM-poh-tense)

Nursing Process Category: Assessment

Incident Report
(IN-sid-ent REE-port)

Nursing Process Category: All

Incontinence
(in-KON-tih-nense)

Nursing Process Category: Assessment

Impotence is also called *erectile dysfunction,* and is the inability to achieve or maintain an erection.

Impotence *is considered a sexual arousal disorder, which is often treated pharmacologically with phosphodiesterase inhibitors such as sildenafil (Viagra).*

An incident report (also called an *occurrence report*) provides an agency record of an accident or unusual occurrence, and includes such information as the client name, facility name, and complete information about the incident, including the date, time, place, witnesses, and any equipment involved in the incident.

*The person who identifies the accident or unusual occurrence should complete the **incident report.***

Incontinence is the inability or difficulty in restraining the natural evacuations of urine or feces. Causes can be muscular or neurologic in nature and nursing interventions will vary according to the client's individual needs.

*Many older women suffer from **urinary incontinence** due to issues related to mobility or neurologic problems.*

Indication
(IN-dih-KAY-shun)

Nursing Process Category: Assessment

Infant
(IN-fant)

Nursing Process Category: Assessment

Infection Control
(in-FEK-shun kon-TROLL)

Nursing Process Category: Implementation

In pharmacotherapy, an indication is the approved use(s) of a drug.

*In the United States, the U.S. Food and Drug Administration (FDA) approves drugs for a specific **indication**(s).*

An infant is a child from the age of 1 month to 1 year.

*Several reflexes can be seen in the **infant**. One example is the rooting reflex, which is a feeding reflex elicited by touching the infant's cheek, which causes the infant to turn to the side that was touched. This reflex usually disappears by 4 months of age.*

Infection control is concerned with preventing health care–associated infection. Infection control deals with concerns related to the spread, prevention, monitoring/investigation, and management of infection.

*The most effective **infection control** method commonly used in health care settings is hand-washing.*

Inflammatory Bowel Disease (IBD)
(in-FLAM-ah-tor-ee BOW-ul dis-EEZ)

Nursing Process Category: Assessment

Informed Consent
(IN-formed kon-SENT)

Nursing Process Category: Implementation

Inspection
(in-SPECK-shun)

Nursing Process Category: Assessment

Inflammatory bowel disease consists of several chronic inflammatory diseases of the gastrointestinal tract.

*The most common types of **inflammatory bowel disease (IBD)** are Crohn's disease and ulcerative colitis. A diagnosis is typically made with barium studies of the upper and lower GI tract, plus examination of the GI tract with an endoscope.*

Informed consent is a voluntary agreement made by a mentally competent client to receive a course of treatment or a procedure. Consent can only be given after the client receives complete information about the treatment or procedure, including any risks and alternatives to the treatment.

*It is vital that the information be provided to the client by the practitioner who will perform the treatment or procedure. A nurse or other health care provider who obtains **informed consent**, yet is not the provider who performs the procedure, exceeds his or her scope of practice, and may face legal consequences.*

Inspection is a visualization of a client in order to gather information. It is the first step in a physical exam.

*The nurse uses **inspection** to check the client's skin in order to determine any changes in texture, color, and size of moles.*

Intradermal (ID)
(IN-trah-DER-mal)

Nursing Process Category: Implementation

Intramuscular (IM)
(IN-trah-MUSS-kew-lar)

Nursing Process Category: Implementation

Intravenous
(IN-trah-VEE-nuss)

Nursing Process Category: Implementation

Intradermal is a method of parenteral medication administration that involves injecting the medication under the epidermis (into the dermis).

*Medications administered by the **intradermal** method avoid the hepatic first-pass effect and digestive enzymes that impact other methods of medication administration.*

Intramuscular is a method of parenteral medication administration that involves delivering the medication into specific muscles.

*In an **intramuscular** injection, the needle is inserted at a 90-degree angle to the site of administration.*

Intravenous is a method of parenteral medication administration that involves administering medications and fluids directly into the bloodstream, which makes the substances immediately available for use by the body.

*The **intravenous** route of medication administration is used when a very rapid onset of action is desired.*

Large Bowel Obstruction (LBO)
(LARJ BOW-ul ahb-STRUK-shun)

Nursing Process Category: Assessment

Leukemia
(lew-KEEM-ee-ah)

Nursing Process Category: Assessment

Lifestyle Choices
(LIFE-sty-ull CHOY-sez)

Nursing Process Category: All

A large bowel obstruction (LBO) is an emergency condition that involves a blockage of the large intestine. Common symptoms include abdominal distention, abdominal cramping, nausea, and vomiting.

*The nurse assesses the client with a **large bowel obstruction (LBO)** for history of bowel movements, flatus, constipation, and symptoms of LBO.*

Leukemia is a class of blood-specific cancers that exist in bone marrow. The cancer depletes blood cells, which causes anemia, infection, hemorrhage, and/or death.

*When administering chemotherapy to a client with **leukemia,** the nurse must be meticulous with oral, skin, and rectal care of the client.*

Lifestyle choices include a client's way of living, which includes patterns of behavior and living conditions that are often influenced by social, cultural, and personal characteristics.

*Lack of exercise and overeating are examples of **lifestyle choices** that cause a higher risk of health conditions such as heart disease and diabetes.*

Loss
(LAWSS)

Nursing Process Category: Assessment

Lung Cancer
(LUNG KAN-serr)

Nursing Process Category: Assessment

Lymphoma
(lim-PHO-mah)

Nursing Process Category: Assessment

Loss is an actual, perceived, or potential situation in which something of value changes or becomes unavailable.

*The nurse counsels clients during all stages of responses to **loss**, including grief, bereavement, and mourning.*

Lung cancer is a particularly deadly form of cancer that is present in the lungs, and includes squamous cell carcinoma, adenocarcinoma, and small and large cell carcinoma.

*The nurse assesses a client's risk for **lung cancer** by obtaining the client's smoking history, as well as any exposure to second-hand smoke or carcinogenic industrial and air pollutants.*

Lymphoma is a cancer (malignant neoplasm) of the lymphocytes, a type of white blood cell. It includes Hodgkin's and non-Hodgkin's lymphoma.

*The nurse recognizes that **lymphoma** is classified in stages, from stage I (localized) to stage IV (extensive involvement to areas such as the bone marrow).*

Malabsorption Syndrome
(mal-ab-SORB-shun SIN-drome)

Nursing Process Category: Assessment

Manager
(MAN-ih-jer)

Nursing Process Category: Implementation

Maslow's Hierarchy of Needs
(MAZ-lows HIGH-err-arr-kee of needz)

*Nursing Process Category: Assessment,
Planning, and Implementation*

Vocabulary

Malabsorption syndrome involves ineffective utilization (absorption) of nutrients from the intestinal tract. It may be associated with certain diseases that affect the intestinal mucosa, such as celiac disease or infections.

*The nurse is aware that the client with **malabsorption syndrome** is at risk for nutrient deficiencies.*

The manager is one of the major functions of nursing. As manager, the nurse organizes, supervises, and directs the care of his or her client. Specific functions can include ensuring that diagnostic tests are scheduled and the client's needs are met.

*The nurse is assigned to provide care to five clients. The nurse must **manage** all the activities (assessments, medication administration, wound care, etc.) involved in the care of his clients.*

Maslow's hierarchy of needs is a theoretical framework that ranks human needs into five levels according to how essential they are to survival; these levels include physiologic, safety and security, love and belonging, self-esteem, and self-actualization. It is based on the work of theorist Abraham Maslow, and nurses use this framework as a guide in promoting the health of clients.

*The nurse understands that clients in the highest level of **Maslow's hierarchy of needs**, the self-actualization level, are aware of and comfortable with their potential, abilities, and qualities. For a client to reach this level, all levels of Maslow's hierarchy of needs must be adequately met.*

Medication Administration "Rights"
(med-ee-CAY-shun ad-min-iss-TRAY-shun RITES)

Nursing Process Category: Implementation

Meningitis
(MEN-in-jy-tiss)

Nursing Process Category: Assessment

Menopause
(MEN-oh-paws)

Nursing Process Category: Assessment

There are six medication administration "rights" that form the basis for safe medication administration. They include: right client, right medication, right dose, right route of administration, right time of delivery, and right documentation. The rights also may include the client's right to refuse, the right assessment, and the right evaluation.

*One of the ways that the nurse can implement the **medication administration rights** is to check the drug before administering it to the client.*

Meningitis is a viral, bacterial, fungal, or mycobacterial infection of the membrane that surrounds the brain, the meninges. Symptoms include fever, chills, headache, stiff neck, altered mental status, and vomiting.

*The nurse recognizes that the CDC recommends the meningococcal vaccine be administered to children beginning at the age of 2 years, for protection from **meningitis.***

Menopause is the permanent cessation of menses, the menstrual cycle in a woman.

*The nurse can assist women in adjusting to the physiologic and psychologic changes that occur during **menopause.***

Mitral Stenosis
(MY-trall sten-OH-siss)

Nursing Process Category: Assessment

Multiple Sclerosis (MS)
(MULL-tih-pull skler-OH-siss)

Nursing Process Category: Assessment

Myasthenia Gravis (MG)
(my-as-THEE-nee-ah GRAH-viss)

Nursing Process Category: Assessment

Mitral stenosis is a narrowing of the mitral valve of the heart, which causes an obstruction of blood flow.

*The nurse assesses the client's history of rheumatic carditis (also known as rheumatic fever), which is known to cause **mitral stenosis.***

Multiple sclerosis is a degenerative disease of the central nervous system characterized by demyelination of neurons.

*The nurse recognizes that common symptoms of **multiple sclerosis** include progressive muscle weakness, visual disturbances, mood alterations, and cognitive deficits.*

Myasthenia gravis is an autoimmune motor disorder caused by acetylcholine receptor abnormalities, which creates muscular fatigue.

*The nurse understands that in clients with **myasthenia gravis (MG),** the most common muscles affected are the eyes, muscles of mastication, and pharyngeal muscles.*

Myocardial Infarction (MI)
(MY-oh-kar-dee-all in-FARK-shun)

Nursing Process Category: Assessment

Neonate
(NEE-oh-nate)

Nursing Process Category: All

Nosocomial Infection
(NO-so-comb-ee-all in-FEK-shun)

Nursing Process Category: Assessment

Also known as a *heart attack*, a myocardial infarction (MI) occurs when the vessels that supply blood to the heart become occluded, and a portion of myocardial tissue becomes necrotic and dies due to the lack of blood supply to the tissue.

*The client presents to the emergency department with chest pain that radiates to the jaw, nausea, and sweating, and is diagnosed with, and treated for, a **myocardial infarction.***

A neonate is an infant from birth to the end of the first month of life.

*The nurse recognizes that the basic task for the **neonate** is to adjust to the environment outside the uterus (the extrauterine environment), which includes breathing, sleep, sucking, eating, swallowing, digestion, and elimination.*

A nosocomial infection is an infection associated with the delivery of health care services in a health care facility, and the infection can arise either during the client's stay or after discharge from the facility.

*One of the most common **nosocomial infections** is urinary tract infection due to improper catheterization techniques.*

Nursing Diagnosis
(NUR-sing dye-ag-NOH-siss)

Nursing Process Category: Diagnosis

Nursing Intervention
(NUR-sing in-ter-VEN-shun)

Nursing Process Category: Implementation

Nursing Process
(NUR-ing PROH-sess)

Nursing Process Category: All

Nursing diagnosis is the second step in the nursing process. It is a statement (or statements) that describes an actual or potential response to a health problem that the nurse is licensed and competent to treat.

*A client with symptoms of diabetes insipidus is admitted to the hospital for evaluation and treatment of the condition. An appropriate **nursing diagnosis** that the nurse should consider for the client is based on an understanding of this condition.*

A nursing intervention is the primary component of the implementation stage of the nursing process, and is any treatment that a nurse performs based on clinical judgment and knowledge to enhance client outcomes.

*An important part of implementing a **nursing intervention** is for the nurse to explain to the client the intervention that will be performed, what the client can expect to feel and do during the intervention, and the expected outcome of the intervention.*

The nursing process is a series of steps or acts that leads to accomplishment of a goal. The purpose of the nursing process is to provide individualized, holistic, and efficient care to clients by identifying client needs, determining priorities, establishing nursing care plans and interventions, and evaluating nursing care. The nursing process includes five steps: assessment, nursing diagnosis, planning, implementation, and evaluation.

*Using the **nursing process,** the nurse develops a plan of care for his or her client.*

Nutritional Care
(noo-TRISH-un-al kair)

Nursing Process Category: Implementation

Nutritional Needs
(new-TRISH-in-ul NEEDZ)

Nursing Process Category: All

Obesity
(oh-BEESE-ih-tee)

Nursing Process Category: Assessment

Nutritional care involves the use of nutritional substances and procedures to ensure the proper intake and assimilation of nutriments, especially for the ill client. Depending on the client needs, nutritional requirements may be provided by oral meals, tube feeding, or parenteral hyperalimentation.

*The client cannot eat due to surgery on his throat. Because it was anticipated he would have problems, a feeding tube was placed prior to surgery so that he could receive **nutritional care.***

Nutritional needs refer to a client's need for the basic building blocks of energy, protein, carbohydrates, and fat. These needs change depending on the client's age and health status.

*During the assessment stage of the nursing process, the nurse determines the client's **nutritional needs** based on the client's health status.*

Obesity is a condition of overnutrition, and is diagnosed when a person's body mass index (BMI) is greater than 30 kg/m^2.

*The client's BMI is determined to be 41 kg/m^2. The nurse recognizes that the client's **obesity** puts stress on body organs and predisposes the client to hypertension, diabetes, and other health issues.*

Objective Data
(ahb-JEK-tiv DAH-tah)

Nursing Process Category: Assessment and Evaluation

Older Adult
(OL-derr ah-DULT)

Nursing Process Category: All

Oral
(OH-rall)

Nursing Process Category: All

Objective data is information the nurse or other health care professional gathers about a client through observation, smell, touch, or hearing; it is usually obtained during physical examination. Information is measurable and is also referred to as *signs* or *overt data.*

*A blood pressure (BP) of 110/60 mm Hg and apical pulse of 80 are some of the **objective data** collected by the nurse during the client assessment.*

An older adult (also called an elder) is someone who is 65 years of age and older. Older adults comprise the fastest-growing age group in the United States.

*In many cultures, such as the Chinese, Native American, Vietnamese, and Korean cultures, the **older adult** is held in high esteem and age is viewed as an asset rather than a liability.*

Oral refers to the mouth, including the cheeks, tongue, teeth, gums, and mucosa. In pharmacotherapy, *oral* refers to administering a medication by mouth, which is an enteral form of medication administration.

***Oral** hygiene, or the care of the teeth and gums, is an important part of health maintenance.*

Osteoarthritis
(OSS-tee-oh-ar-THRY-tiss)

Nursing Process Category: Assessment

Osteoporosis
(OSS-tee-oh-pore-OH-siss)

Nursing Process Category: Assessment

Outcome(s)
(OUT-kum)

Nursing Process Category: Planning

Osteoarthritis is a type of arthritis in which the cartilage in synovial joints and vertebrae progressively deteriorates.

*The client is a middle-aged man who has played recreational football for most of his life, and is experiencing symptoms of **osteoarthritis** in one knee as a result of the overuse and abuse of the knee joint.*

Osteoporosis is a loss of bone density that may lead to spontaneous fractures (pathologic fractures).

*The nurse assists a client in planning a regimen of exercise, including weight-bearing exercise and nutrition, to help slow the loss of bone density due to **osteoporosis.***

An outcome, also referred to as a *desired outcome*, is a desired result(s) that is specific in nature. In nursing, client outcomes are described in terms of measurable, observable client responses used to evaluate whether goals have been met.

*The client goal is to be free of pain. A **desired outcome** associated with this goal is that the client will state that his pain is a 0 on the pain scale of 1–10, 30 minutes after receiving pain medication.*

Oxygenate
(OX-ih-juh-NAYT)

Oxygenation
(OX-ih-juh-NAY-shun)

Nursing Process Category: Implementation

Pain
(peyn)

Nursing Process Category: Assessment

Pain Relief Measures
(PAYNE ree-LEEF MEH-zures)

Nursing Process Category: Planning, Implementation, and Evaluation

Oxygenation is the process of treating or combining with oxygen.

*Clients who do not have enough oxygen in their bloodstream (PO_2) may need **oxygenation** therapy by way of a nasal cannula mask.*

Pain is a subjective, unpleasant feeling of physical, mental, or emotional suffering or distress that is usually due to injury or illness. Pain is a cardinal symptom of inflammation. Responses vary from individual to individual and can be acute or chronic in nature.

*Many conditions, such as rheumatoid arthritis, cause noxious stimulation of sensory nerve endings and create severe **pain**.*

Also called *pain management*, pain relief measures are nursing interventions or client self-directed methods to reduce pain. Pain relief measures can be pharmacologic (involving administration of medications to relieve pain) or nonpharmacologic such as massage or the use of other diversional techniques.

*For **pain relief measures** that the client implements in the home setting, the nurse teaches the client to keep a pain diary to monitor pain onset, intensity, location, and relief measures.*

Palpate
(PAL-pate)

Palpation
(pal-PAY-shun)

Nursing Process Category: Assessment

Pancreatitis
(PAN-kree-ah-TYE-tiss)

Nursing Process Category: Assessment

Parenteral
(pare-EN-terr-all)

Nursing Process Category: Implementation

Palpation is a method of feeling with the hands during a physical examination. The nurse touches and feels the client's body to examine the size, consistency, texture, location, and tenderness of an organ or body part.

*The nurse uses **palpation** when determining a client's pulse.*

Pancreatitis is literally the inflammation of the pancreas; symptoms include severe upper abdominal pain, nausea, and vomiting. There are two types of pancreatitis, acute and chronic.

*The nurse recognizes that the most common cause of acute **pancreatitis** is gallstones, and the most common cause of chronic **pancreatitis** is excessive alcohol consumption (though the latter can also contribute to acute pancreatitis).*

Parenteral refers to a method of medication administration by routes other than oral or topical, and includes intradermal (skin layers), subcutaneous, intramuscular (muscle), and intravenous (vein) routes.

*The nurse must strictly use aseptic techniques during **parenteral** medication administration due to the potential for introducing pathogenic microbes directly into the client's blood or tissues.*

Parkinson's Disease
(PARK-in-sons dis-EEZ)

Nursing Process Category: Assessment

Peptic Ulcer
(PEP-tik ULL-sir)

Nursing Process Category: Assessment

Percussion
(per-KUH-shun)

Nursing Process Category: Assessment

Parkinson's disease is a neurologic condition that involves the misfiring of nerve cells due to damaged or degenerated dopamine-producing brain cells.

*The nurse assesses that the client's symptoms of **Parkinson's disease** have become worse since the previous visit, and there is now postural instability and impaired balance and coordination.*

A peptic ulcer (also called *peptic ulcer disease [PUD]*) is a mucosal erosion of the lining of the stomach, duodenum (upper small intestine), or esophagus. The ulcer occurs from mucosal damage due to excess stomach acid.

*The nurse understands that the most common cause of **peptic ulcer** is infection with the bacterium Helicobacter pylori (H. pylori).*

Percussion is a method of tapping body parts with fingers, hands, or small instruments as part of a physical examination with the purpose to evaluate the size, consistency, borders, and presence or absence of fluid in body organs.

*The nurse uses **percussion** to check the client's abdomen in order to assess organ and tissue density.*

Peripheral Vascular Disease (PVD)
(pur-IF-ur-all VASS-kew-lar dis-EEZ)

Nursing Process Category: Assessment

Pharmacotherapy
(FAR-ma-ko-THAIR-ah-pee)

Nursing Process Category: Implementation

Planning
(PLAN-ing)

Nursing Process Category: Planning

Peripheral vascular disease (PVD) (also called *peripheral artery disease [PAD]*) involves a narrowing or complete obstruction of the vessels that carry blood to peripheral areas, which include areas outside the chest such as the arms, legs, feet, or even the stomach or kidneys.

*The nurse recognizes that cigarette smoking is the most common modifiable cause of **peripheral vascular disease (PVD)**.*

Pharmacotherapy is the treatment or prevention of disease with the use of drugs.

*The nurse's primary role in **pharmacotherapy** is client education and monitoring and evaluating the effects of the medication.*

Planning is the third step in the nursing process, and is a method used to prioritize nursing diagnosis and organize interventions in order to achieve the goals of client care. It includes the development of individualized client care plans.

*When **planning** a client's care, the nurse and client should work together to determine the goals and outcomes.*

Pneumonia
(NEW-moan-yah)

Nursing Process Category: Assessment

Pneumothorax
(NEW-moe-THOR-ax)

Nursing Process Category: Assessment

Postoperative Care
(post-OPP-err-ah-tiv KAIR)

Nursing Process Category: Implementation

Pneumonia is the inflammation of the lining of the lungs that is usually caused by infection with bacteria, viruses, or another pathogenic organism.

*One of the tests used to determine the treatment for **pneumonia** is the Gram stain sputum test.*

Pneumothorax is a collection of air in the pleural cavity of the lung, which enters as a result of perforation through the chest wall from injury or through the pleura.

*Chest tubes are inserted into the pleural cavity to restore negative pressure as a result of **pneumothorax.***

Postoperative care by the nurse encompasses interventions provided for the client during the period following a surgical procedure. Postoperative care interventions include pain management, respiratory monitoring, infection control, and teaching for home care.

*To follow the nursing process in providing **postoperative care**, the nurse implements any postoperative orders from the surgeon or primary care provider.*

Potential Problems
(po-TEN-shul PROB-lum)

Nursing Process Category: Nursing Diagnosis

Pregnancy
(PREG-nan-see)

Nursing Process Category: Assessment

Preoperative Care
(pree-OPP-er-ah-tiv KAIR)

Nursing Process Category: Implementation

A potential problem is a problem that is capable of becoming real and current, of becoming a potential danger to client safety.

*The client has just had surgery on her left hip. Even though she is not currently showing any signs of an infection, because of the nature of the surgery, she has the **potential problem** of infection. On the nursing care plan, this problem is addressed with the nursing diagnosis of "Risk for Infection."*

Pregnancy is the condition of containing a developing embryo or fetus within the body after conception. The typical length of pregnancy is about 280 days, or 9 months.

*The nurse plays an important role in teaching the pregnant woman about the physiologic changes of **pregnancy**, as well as prenatal care and ways to minimize the discomforts of **pregnancy**.*

Preoperative care encompasses the nursing actions performed for a client who will undergo a surgical procedure (inpatient or outpatient), and includes client assessment, identifying any actual or potential health problems, and teaching to prepare the client and family mentally and physically for surgery.

*As part of **preoperative care**, the nurse explains to the client and family individual therapies ordered by the primary care provider, such as the insertion of a urinary catheter.*

Preschool Age (Child)
(PREE-skool AGE)

Nursing Process Category: All

Prevent
(pree-VENT)
Prevention
(pree-VENT-shun)

Nursing Process Category: Implementation

Prioritize
(pry-OR-ih-tize)

Nursing Process Category: Planning

Preschool age is a period of development in children who are between the ages of 4 and 5 years.

*Because a child at the **preschool age** is spending more time away from parents in settings such as school and daycare, it is important to teach the child simple safety rules, such as crossing the street or bicycle and playground safety.*

Prevention (to prevent) is to keep or avert something from occurring, usually something of negative consequence.

*The nurse is assigned to give medications to six clients on a medical unit starting at 9 a.m. She **prevents** any errors from occurring by following the six rights of drug administration.*

To prioritize is to do something according to what is determined to be highest or higher in importance.

*Nurses must learn to **prioritize** the care they give to their clients because of the many demands placed on nurses.*

Prostate Cancer

(PROSS-tate KAN-serr)

Nursing Process Category: Assessment

Psoriasis

(sore-EYE-ah-siss)

Nursing Process Category: Assessment

Quality Assurance (QA)

(KWAL-ih-tee ah-SURE-anse)

Nursing Process Category: All

Prostate cancer is a malignant tumor of the prostate gland, and symptoms include difficult urination, urinary hesitancy or frequency, urinary stream reduction, and excessive urination at night (nocturia).

*Screening for **prostate cancer** includes prostate-specific antigen (PSA) tests as well as annual digital rectal examinations for men beginning at age 50.*

Psoriasis is a painful, chronic, inflammatory disease of the skin characterized by red lesions covered with silvery scales on the epidermis.

*The nurse assists the client to identify and reduce or eliminate stressors that may exacerbate **psoriasis,** such as emotional stress, infection, and cold weather.*

Quality assurance (QA) is an ongoing process that evaluates and promotes excellence in the provision of health care to groups of clients, and includes evaluating the following components of care: structure, process, and outcome.

*One key part of **quality assurance** is the evaluative process, which examines how care was given to the clients and determines whether the care was relevant to the client's needs.*

Recommended Dietary Intake (RDI)
(REK-oh-men-did DIE-ih-tare-ee IN-tayk)

Nursing Process Category: Planning and Implementation

Referral
(ref-ERR-al)

Nursing Process Category: Implementation

Regular Diet
(REG-you-lar DYE-it)

Nursing Process Category: Implementation

Also called *reference dietary intake*, the recommended dietary intake (RDI) is the government-recommended amounts of vitamins, minerals, and other nutrients. More specifically, the RDI refers to the Dietary Reference Intake (DRI) tables published by the Committee on the Scientific Evaluation of Dietary Reference Intakes of the Institute of Medicine. The DRI tables contain four sets of reference values, including the estimated average requirements (EARs), recommended dietary allowances (RDAs), adequate intakes (AIs), and tolerable upper intake levels (ULs).

The food labels required by the U.S. Food and Drug Administration (FDA), called Nutrition Facts, is where consumers most commonly learn **recommended dietary intake (RDI)** *information.*

Referral is the process of sending a client to another health care provider for consultation or service, and is often done by a primary care provider to a specialized care provider.

A 59-year-old client recently diagnosed with Parkinson's disease questions the nurse about a **referral** *to a geriatrician, and the nurse explains that the geriatrician specializes in diseases that usually affect older adults.*

A regular diet is a nonrestricted, nontherapeutic diet that consists of all food groups, and is a well-balanced diet necessary to maintain health for hospitalized clients. It is also called a *normal, standard, or house diet.*

A **regular diet** *typically follows the dietary guidelines established by the U.S. Department of Agriculture (USDA) to ensure that the client receives the essential nutrients needed for recovery.*

Renal Failure
(REE-nall FAIL-yur)

Nursing Process Category: Assessment

Rest
(REST)

Nursing Process Category: Implementation

Rheumatoid Arthritis
(ROO-mah-toyd arr-THRY-tiss)

Nursing Process Category: Assessment

Renal failure (also known as *kidney failure*) is characterized by inadequate functioning of the kidneys, and may be temporary, partial, acute, or chronic in nature.

The 77-year-old female client was diagnosed with **renal failure** *and required the initiation of dialysis.*

Rest—which is a period of inactivity, relaxation, or sleep—is essential to health. When deprived of sleep, clients can become agitated, irritable, and possibly depressed. Adequate rest helps to restore normal body functions.

It is the responsibility of nurses to create an environment where their clients can receive the **rest** *they need.*

Rheumatoid arthritis is a chronic, systemic autoimmune disease characterized by swelling, pain, morning stiffness, and sometimes deformity in multiple joints.

The 56-year-old female client who is experiencing chronic pain from **rheumatoid arthritis** *is referred to the rheumatologist for routine pain control assessment.*

Safety
(SAFE-ty)

Nursing Process Category: All

Safety Device
(SAYF-tee DEE-vice)

Nursing Process Category: Implementation

Schizophrenia
(SKITS-oh-FREN-ee-ah)

Nursing Process Category: Assessment

Safety is the ability of people to prevent, and protect themselves from, accident or injury.

*The nurse ensures client **safety** by assessing the client's age and development, lifestyle and home environment, mobility and health status, sensory-perceptual alterations, emotional state, and cognitive awareness.*

A safety device is a product used to prevent injury in the home or health care facility setting, and includes smoke and carbon monoxide detectors, electrical outlet covers, or a bed or chair exit safety monitoring device that triggers an audio alarm when the client attempts to get out of bed or a chair.

*The choice of a **safety device** is dependent upon the client's developmental stage, physical abilities, and specific health needs.*

Schizophrenia is a mental disorder characterized by abnormal thoughts and thought processes, such as delusions, hallucinations, and disorganized speech and behavior as well as social withdrawal.

***Schizophrenia** is frequently treated with drugs that act on dopamine receptors in the brain; such drugs are associated with significant side effects that require careful monitoring.*

School Age (Child)
(SKOOL AGE)

Nursing Process Category: All

Scope of Practice
(SKOPE of PRAK-tiss)

Nursing Process Category: All

Security Needs
(see-KUR-ih-tee NEEDZ)

Nursing Process Category: Assessment, Planning, and Implementation

School age is a period of development for a child between the ages of 6 and 12 years. The school-age period ends with the onset of puberty.

*The nurse performs a developmental assessment of the **school-age** child, and includes physical, motor, and psychosocial developmental assessments such as physical growth, motor skills, and interaction with parents and peers.*

Scope of practice is the range of health care–related activities and services that a health care professional is educated, and licensed or certified, to provide. Specific guidelines of practice are described and regulated by a state regulatory board.

*To safely provide care, the registered nurse must follow the guidelines indicated in the nurse's **scope of practice**.*

Security needs are part of the basic needs of every person, and reflect the need to be safe (freedom from danger, fear, or anxiety) in the physical environment as well as in relationships.

*A person's needs are interrelated, which means that one need is often dependent on another need. For example, a respiratory obstruction can threaten the need for oxygen (a physiologic need), which markedly alters **security needs**.*

Sickle Cell Disease
(SIK-ill CELL dis-EEZ)

Nursing Process Category: Assessment

Signs
(SIGHNZ)

Nursing Process Category: Assessment

Skin Cancer
(SKIN KAN-ser)

Nursing Process Category: Assessment

Sickle cell disease (also called *sickle cell anemia*) is an autosomal recessive blood disorder in which the red blood cells become sickled, or crescent shaped, which affects the cells' ability to pass through small blood vessels. The sickled red blood cells block vessels and impede the flow of blood to various tissues.

*The main goals of **sickle cell disease** treatment are to relieve pain, and to prevent infections, eye damage, and stroke.*

Signs, commonly known as objective information (data), are overt in nature and are detectable by the observer or can be measured by acceptable tests. Signs can be seen, heard, felt, or smelled. Examples of signs are pulse rate and lung sounds.

*The nurse assesses the following **signs** from the client: temperature of 99°F, pulse rate of 86, and a respiration rate of 20.*

Skin cancer is a term that encompasses various types of malignant neoplasms that occur in the skin, including basal cell carcinoma, squamous cell carcinoma, and melanoma.

*Excessive exposure to ultraviolet light (sun exposure) is associated with all types of **skin cancer**.*

Sodium-Restricted Diet
(SOH-dee-um ree-STRIK-ted DYE-it)

Nursing Process Category: Implementation

Soft Diet
(SOFT DYE-it)

Nursing Process Category: Implementation

Spinal Tap
(SPY-nall TAPP)

Nursing Process Category: Implementation

A sodium-restricted diet (also called a *low-salt diet*) is a therapeutic diet for clients who require low-sodium foods and drinks, and is often prescribed to clients with cardiac and renal disease.

*The 47-year-old male client with newly diagnosed hypertension is prescribed a **sodium-restricted diet,** and the nurse assists in reinforcing instruction from the care provider as well as the dietitian.*

A soft diet involves modifying a diet so that all food is of a soft consistency in order to make the food more easily chewed and digested. This diet is low in fiber and contains very few uncooked foods.

*The client with difficulty chewing and swallowing is prescribed a **soft diet,** and the first meal consists of scrambled eggs, spinach, and oatmeal.*

Also called a *lumbar puncture*, a spinal tap is a procedure in which cerebrospinal fluid (CSF) is withdrawn through a needle. The needle is inserted into the subarachnoid space between the third and fourth (or fourth and fifth) lumbar vertebrae.

*After a **spinal tap,** the nurse assists the client to a dorsal recumbent (or supine) position with one head pillow; the client remains in this position from 1 to 12 hours, depending on orders from the primary care provider.*

Spiritual Need
(SPEER-it-you-al NEED)

Nursing Process Category: All

Standard Precautions
(STAND-ard PREE-caw-shuns)

Nursing Process Category: Implementation

Standard(s)
(STAN-dard)

Nursing Process Category: All

A spiritual need is a component of growth and development, and reflects the person's need to understand his or her relationship with the universe and the direction and meaning of life.

A person's **spiritual need** *may be expressed by actively participating in a particular faith tradition and interacting with others who are living a particular faith tradition.*

Standard precautions are measures taken to prevent the spread of infections or potentially infectious microorganisms to health care professionals, clients, and facility visitors. The Centers for Disease Control (CDC) issues guidelines for standard precautions for health care facilities.

An example of **standard precautions** *is for the nurse to wear personal protective equipment (PPE) such as a mask, eye protection, or a face shield if splashes or sprays of body fluids, blood, secretions, or excretions are expected.*

Standards are morals, ethics, or rules usually established by an authority as acceptable. In nursing, standards can be found in various codes of ethics and organizational policy and procedure manuals.

Nurses are expected to follow the **standards** *of care established by the hospital where they are employed.*

Stress Management
(STRESS MAN-aj-ment)

Nursing Process Category: Implementation

Subcutaneous
(SUB-cue-TANE-ee-uss)

Nursing Process Category: Implementation

Subjective Data
(sub-JEK-tiv DAH-tah)

Nursing Process Category: Assessment

Stress management is the use of any measure to reduce or eliminate stress or anxiety. Such measures can include relaxation techniques, counseling, exercise, and support groups.

It is essential for both nurses and clients to develop successful **stress management** *techniques to prevent the negative consequences of stress and anxiety.*

Subcutaneous is a parenteral route of medication administration that involves delivering the medication to the deepest layers of the skin.

Several body sites that are ideal for **subcutaneous** *injections are the outer aspect of the upper arm, the middle two-thirds of the anterior thigh, and the upper dorsogluteal and ventrogluteal areas.*

Subjective data, also called *symptoms* or *overt data*, is information that is apparent only to the person affected, such as the client's sensations, feelings, values, beliefs, and perception of his or her personal health status.

An example of **subjective data** *is when a client states, "I get short of breath when walking after climbing only a few stairs."*

Supervision
(SUP-err-VISH-un)

Nursing Process Category: Implementation

Surgical Asepsis
(SURJ-ik-al ay-SEP-siss)

Nursing Process Category: Implementation

Symptoms
(SYM-tumz)

Nursing Process Category: Assessment

Supervision is the process of watching and directing another's actions, such as the nurse supervising the tasks performed by unlicensed assistive personnel (UAP).

*The nurse may be responsible for the **supervision** of other health care workers such as licensed practical nurses (LPN) and nursing assistants.*

Surgical asepsis, also called sterile technique, encompasses practices that keep an area or object free from all microorganisms and spores. It is used for any procedure that involves the sterile areas of the body, such as insertion of a catheter.

*The nurse uses **surgical asepsis** when preparing the client for any surgical procedure.*

Symptoms, commonly known as *subjective information* (data), are apparent only to the person affected and can be described only by that person. A symptom is an indication of a condition. Examples of symptoms can include pain, itching, and feelings of anxiety.

*Following surgery for removal of a brain tumor, the client complains of a severe headache. The nurse recognizes this **symptom** is probably the result of the surgery.*

Syphilis
(SIFF-ill-iss)

Nursing Process Category: Assessment

Systemic Lupus Erythematosus (SLE)
(siss-TEM-ik LOO-puss air-ITH-eem-ah-TOW-siss)

Nursing Process Category: Assessment

Teaching
(TEE-ching)
Teach
(TEECH)

Nursing Process Category: Implementation

Syphilis is a sexually transmitted infection (STI) caused by the *Treponema pallidum* spirochete; a small number of syphilis infections may also occur during pregnancy.

*The 38-year-old male client presents with a chancre on his penis as well as a low-grade fever and inflamed lymph glands, and is diagnosed with **syphilis.***

Systemic lupus erythematosus (SLE), often called just *lupus*, is an autoimmune disease in which acute and chronic inflammation is present in various tissues of the body, such as the heart, joints, skin, and nervous system. Those with lupus experience periods of illness, called *flares*, that alternate with periods of remission.

*The nurse assigns the nursing diagnosis of Disturbed Body Image to the client with **systemic lupus erythematosus (SLE)** due to the client's expressed negative feelings about her body related to SLE-related rash and mottled erythema of hands and face.*

Teaching is the process of providing instruction to someone in need, such as a client. Teaching can be done through a variety of methods such as discussion and demonstration.

*The nurse makes plans to prepare the client for the T3 (triiodothyronine) and T4 (thyroxin) uptake test. The client **teaching** plan should include that the client will need to have her blood drawn regularly.*

Terminal Illness
(TURR-mih-nil ILL-niss)

Nursing Process Category: Assessment

Therapeutic
(thair-uh-PEW-tik)

Nursing Process Category: All

Therapeutic Communication
(thair-ih-PEW-tik kah-MYOON-ih-KAY-shun)

Nursing Process Category: All

Terminal illness is an unhealthy condition that causes the end of life, or having an illness where there is no reasonable chance of survival.

*Some clients with a **terminal illness** choose to receive palliative care by a hospice nurse.*

The term *therapeutic* means "to be beneficial." Therefore, all actions or treatments are directed toward the client's benefit.

*The nurse uses **therapeutic** communication techniques to help the client better understand his treatment options.*

Therapeutic communication is a way for nurses to interact with clients to promote understanding and establish a constructive relationship.

*An example of **therapeutic communication** is for the nurse to use open-ended questions when speaking with the client, such as, "Please describe your pain."*

Therapeutic Diet
(thair-ih-PEW-tik DYE-it)

Nursing Process Category: Implementation

Toddler
(TODD-lerr)

Nursing Process Category: All

Topical
(TOP-ik-al)

Nursing Process Category: Implementation

A therapeutic diet, also called a *special diet*, is one that is prescribed for a client with a specific health concern in order to either treat the condition or prevent exacerbation of the symptoms.

*The 36-year-old male client with newly diagnosed type II diabetes mellitus is prescribed a **therapeutic diet** to help him control his blood sugar levels.*

A toddler is a child between the ages of 1 to 3 years, and development during this time spans from having no voluntary control to being able to walk and speak.

*Long before a **toddler** can form words into sentences, he or she can understand words and follow directions.*

"Topical" refers to a method of medication administration in which a medication is applied to the skin or the membrane of the eye, ear, nose, respiratory tract, urinary tract, vagina, and rectum. Topical drugs produce a local (versus systemic) effect.

*A transdermal nitroglycerin patch is an example of a **topical** route of medication administration.*

Total Parenteral Nutrition (TPN)
(TOE-tall pair-EN-terr-all new-TRISH-un)

Nursing Process Category: Implementation

Urinary Hesitancy
(YOOR-uh-nair-ee HEZ-ih-TUHN-see)

Nursing Process Category: Assessment

Urinary Frequency
(YOOR-uh-nair-ee FREE-kwuhn-see)

Nursing Process Category: Assessment

Also referred to as *hyperalimentation,* total parenteral nutrition helps clients whose nutritional needs cannot be met through enteral nutrition, which is the administration of nutritional supplements via the gastrointestinal tract either orally or through a feeding tube. Parenteral nutrition is administration of nutritional supplements by means of IV infusion, either by peripheral vein or central vein.

*The hypertonic nutrition solution used in **total parenteral nutrition** contains amino acids, lipids, carbohydrate, electrolytes, vitamins, and minerals and is administered through an infusion pump for precise monitoring.*

Urinary hesitancy is difficulty in starting or maintaining a urinary stream.

*Many men with benign prostatic hypertrophy (BPH), an enlarged prostate, have a problem with **urinary hesitancy.***

Urinary frequency is a greater than normal urge to urinate without an increase in the daily volume. Bladder inflammation due to infection or a diminished bladder capacity due to structural abnormalities can cause this condition.

*The client came to the clinic complaining of **urinary frequency** and was diagnosed with a bladder infection.*

Urinary Tract Infection (UTI)
(YOU-rin-air-ee TRAKT in-FEK-shun)

Nursing Process Category: Assessment

Viral Hepatitis (VH)
(VY-rall hep-ah-TITE-iss)

Nursing Process Category: Assessment

Vital Signs
(VYE-til SIGHNZ)

Nursing Process Category: Assessment

A urinary tract infection is an infection of the kidneys, ureters, or bladder by a microorganism, and is a common nosocomial (health care facility-acquired) infection that is often caused by *Escherichia coli*. UTIs occur more often in women due to the shorter urethra and proximity of the urethra to the anal and vaginal areas.

*The nurse provides instructions to a female client who is experiencing a **urinary tract infection (UTI)**, and advises the client to drink eight 8-ounce glasses of water per day to flush bacteria out of the urinary system.*

Viral hepatitis, often called just *hepatitis*, is inflammation of the liver due to infection with one of the hepatitis viruses. The most common hepatitis viruses are types A, B, and C.

*The 49-year-old male client presents with symptoms of jaundice, anorexia, and fatigue and is diagnosed with **viral hepatitis** after blood tests confirm the diagnosis.*

Vital signs are measurements of the following essential body functions: pulse rate, body temperature, respiration, and blood pressure. Vital signs provide information about the health of a person.

*The nurse is responsible for regularly monitoring the **vital signs** of his or her clients to gain knowledge of their general health status.*

Wellness

(WELL-ness)

Nursing Process Category: All

Wellness is a state of well-being, and includes a balance of basic components such as emotional, physical, spiritual, intellectual, occupation, environmental, and social well-being.

*The nurse recognizes that the definition of **wellness** is highly individual and varies from person to person.*

Generic: acetaminophen (ah-seet-ah-MIN-oh-fen)

Brand: Tylenol

Classification(s): Antipyretic; nonnarcotic analgesic

Generic: acyclovir (ah-SYE-kloh-veer)

Brand: Zovirax

Classification(s): Antiviral; antiherpes antiviral

Side Effects: Hepatotoxicity, rare allergic reactions

Nursing Implications and Precautions:

- If client is taking warfarin, monitor for increased risk of bleeding.
- Advise client to limit or avoid alcohol use during therapy.
- Advise client to not use for fever for more than 3 days unless directed by the prescriber.
- Monitor for hepatotoxicity.
- If overdose is suspected, acetylcysteine is the antidote.

Side Effects: Nausea, diarrhea, allergic reaction, malaise

Nursing Implications and Precautions:

- Advise client to take drug for the entire length of time prescribed, even if lesions are healing or disappear.
- Use gloves when applying topical forms of the drug.
- If using liquid forms, shake the bottle well before dispensing.

Generic: albuterol (al-BUE-ter-ahl)

Brand: ProAir HFA, Proventil HFA, Ventolin HFA, VoSpire ER

Classification(s): Bronchodilator (respiratory smooth muscle relaxant); beta-adrenergic agonist

Generic: alendronate (ah-LEN-droh-nate)

Brand: Fosamax

Classification(s): Bone metabolism regulator; bisphosphonate

Side Effects: Paradoxical bronchospasm, increased blood pressure, tachycardia, ECG changes, allergic reactions, nervousness

Nursing Implications and Precautions:

- Administer with caution to clients with cardiovascular disorders such as coronary artery disease, dysrhythmias, or hypertension.

- If using an inhaler, teach client proper use of the device.

- Do not administer with a beta-adrenergic blocker, unless directed by the prescriber.

- If administering with a diuretic, monitor for potential hypokalemia.

- Advise client to take drug 30 minutes prior to anticipated exercise.

- Advise client to notify the prescriber immediately if the drug stops working well or if more doses per day are needed to prevent breathing difficulties.

Side Effects: Diarrhea, constipation, flatulence, nausea, vomiting, headache, metallic taste, musculoskeletal pain, pathologic fractures, osteonecrosis of the jaw

Nursing Implications and Precautions:

- Administer drug with plain water, preferably 1–2 hours before breakfast.

- Ensure that client remains upright for at least 30 minutes after taking drug.

- Advise client to immediately report jaw pain, swelling, loose teeth, or gum infections.

- Do not administer with medicines that contain calcium, aluminum, or magnesium.

- Assess results of periodic bone mineral density tests to ensure effectiveness of therapy.

- Advise client to include adequate amounts of vitamin D and calcium in the diet.

Generic: allopurinol (al-oh-PURE-in-all)

Brand: Zyloprim

Classification(s): Antigout

Side Effects: Nausea, vomiting, drowsiness, malaise, rash, toxic epidermal necrolysis and Stevens-Johnson syndrome (rare), severe hypersensitivity syndrome (rare)

Nursing Implications and Precautions:

- Discontinue therapy and notify the prescriber at first appearance of skin rash or symptoms suggesting an allergic reaction.
- Advise client to immediately report rash, blistering of the skin, or flu symptoms.
- Administer with a full glass of water and ensure fluid intake of least 8–10 glasses per day.

- Advise client to limit or eliminate alcohol intake during therapy.
- Monitor hepatic function tests and assess for possible hepatotoxicity during the early stages of therapy.
- Advise client to avoid driving and other hazardous activities until the effects of the drug are known.

Generic: alprazolam (all-PRAY-zoh-lam)

Brand: Niravam, Xanax

Classification(s): Antianxiety; sedative-hypnotic; benzodiazepine

Side Effects: Dizziness, ataxia, drowsiness, sedation, confusion, dependence, blurred vision, seizures, birth defects (pregnancy Category D)

Nursing Implications and Precautions:

- Advise client to not discontinue the drug abruptly.

- Advise client to avoid driving and other hazardous activities until the effects of the drug are known.

- Do not administer to clients with suicidal ideation.

- Assess for signs of overdose or abuse (confusion, sedation, slurred speech, coma).

- Advise client to store drug in a safe place, away from children or those who may take the drug for recreational purposes.

- Advise the female client to immediately notify the prescriber of known or suspected pregnancy.

- Advise client to limit or eliminate alcohol use during therapy because this may cause excessive drowsiness.

- Do not administer drug with grapefruit juice.

- Advise the client taking alprazolam to allow the tablet to dissolve in the mouth without chewing or swallowing whole.

- Use caution when administering other CNS depressants concurrently with alprazolam due to the potential for excessive sedation.

Generic: amitriptyline (am-ih-TRIP-till-een)

Brand: Elavil

Classification(s): Antidepressant, tricyclic

Generic: amlodipine (am-LOW-dih-peen)

Brand: Norvasc

Classification(s): Antihypertensive; antianginal; calcium channel blocker

Side Effects: Suicidal ideation, dry mouth, sedation, confusion, orthostatic hypotension, urinary retention, tachycardia, drowsiness, blurred vision, constipation, neuroleptic malignant syndrome (rare)

Nursing Implications and Precautions:

- Monitor for worsening depression and suicidal ideation.
- Advise client to avoid driving and other hazardous activities until the effects of the drug are known.
- Advise client to continue taking the drug, even if feeling better.
- Advise client that the drug must be taken several weeks before its full effects are noticed.

- Use with caution in clients with benign prostatic hyperplasia, hepatic impairment, hyperthyroidism, and Parkinson's disease.
- Advise client to move slowly from a lying to a standing position to prevent light-headedness.
- Do not administer this drug to clients taking monoamine oxidase (MAO) inhibitors.

Side Effects: Flushing, hypotension, headache, dizziness, peripheral edema, hepatotoxicity, heart failure, reflex tachycardia

Nursing Implications and Precautions:

- Assess for swelling of hands, feet, and ankles.
- Use with caution in clients with heart failure or hepatic impairment.
- Monitor blood pressure periodically to ensure drug effectiveness.
- Advise client to continue taking the drug, even if symptoms resolve.
- Advise client to stop smoking because tobacco use decreases the effectiveness of the drug.

- Advise client to limit or eliminate alcohol use during therapy.
- Advise client to move slowly from a lying to a standing position to prevent light-headedness.
- Monitor client carefully when beginning therapy or changing doses because this may worsen angina pain or cause a myocardial infarction.

Generic: amoxicillin (ah-mox-ah-SILL-in)

Brand: Amoxil, Trimox

Classification(s): Antibiotic; aminopenicillin

Generic: amphetamine and **dextroamphetamine**
(dex-troh-am-FET-ah-meen)

Brand: Adderall

Classification(s): Anorexiant; cerebral stimulant

Side Effects: Diarrhea, nausea, vomiting, allergic reactions

Nursing Implications and Precautions:

- Assess for history of hypersensitivity to penicillins or other antibiotics.
- Monitor for allergic reactions, including anaphylaxis.
- Monitor for pseudomembranous colitis (severe diarrhea).
- Monitor clients with mononucleosis carefully for skin rashes.
- Advise client to take drug for the entire length of time prescribed, even if symptoms of infection have resolved.

Side Effects: Irritability, insomnia, nervousness, palpitations, anorexia, elevated blood pressure, paranoia, euphoria, hallucinations, tremor, dependence, sudden death (in clients with pre-existing structural cardiac abnormalities or other serious heart conditions)

Nursing Implications and Precautions:

- Monitor for signs of excessive CNS stimulation (irritability, insomnia, nervousness, palpitations, tremor).
- Do not administer to clients taking monoamine oxidase (MAO) inhibitors.
- Use with caution in clients with heart disease, hypertension, hyperthyroidism, diabetes, glaucoma, and bipolar disorder.
- In children, monitor growth and weight during therapy because this drug can suppress long-term growth.
- Advise client to store drug in a safe place, away from children or those who may take the drug for recreational purposes.
- Advise clients taking extended-release forms to swallow the drug whole and not to crush, split, or chew the capsules.
- Assess the cardiovascular status (including family history) of the client prior to starting therapy.
- Use with caution in clients with a history of drug abuse.

Generic: amphotericin B (am-foh-TARE-ah-sin)

Brand: Abelcet, others

Classification(s): Antifungal

Generic: aripiprazole (ar-ih-PIP-rah-zole)

Brand: Abilify

Classification(s): Antipsychotic, atypical; dopamine system stabilizer

Side Effects: Fever and chills, vomiting, anorexia, headache, phlebitis, hearing impairment, nephrotoxicity, electrolyte imbalances, hepatotoxicity

Nursing Implications and Precautions:

- Perform baseline hearing function tests prior to therapy and assess for gradual hearing loss.

- Monitor urine intake/output and laboratory tests of renal function: Discontinue drug if blood urea nitrogen (BUN) exceeds 40 mg/dL or serum creatinine exceeds 3 mg/dL.

- Use caution when administering other nephrotoxic or hepatotoxic drugs during therapy.

- Administer IV drug over 4–6 hours to prevent shock.

- Assess infusion site for extravasation and signs of phlebitis.

Side Effects: Drowsiness, insomnia, changes in blood pressure, agitation, dizziness, headache, nausea, vomiting, stroke, unusual changes in behavior, neuroleptic malignant syndrome (rare), orthostatic hypotension, akathisia

Nursing Implications and Precautions:

- Use with caution in older adult clients with dementia-related psychoses because there is an increased risk of death.

- Monitor for unusual changes in behavior, worsening depression, and suicidal ideation.

- Use with caution in clients with diabetes or seizure disorders.

- Advise client to avoid driving and other hazardous activities until the effects of the drug are known.

- Assess for tardive dyskinesia; discontinue drug and notify prescriber immediately.

- Assess for extrapyramidal symptoms in clients concurrently taking other antipsychotic drugs or lithium.

- Advise client to move slowly from a lying to a standing position to prevent light-headedness.

- Advise client to take drug for the entire length of time prescribed, even if feeling better.

Generic: aspirin (AS-purr-in)

Brand: ASA, many others

Classification(s): Antipyretic; antiplatelet; nonnarcotic analgesic, salicylate

Generic: atenolol (ah-TEN-oh-loll)

Brand: Tenormin

Classification(s): Antihypertensive; beta-adrenergic antagonist

Side Effects: Heartburn, gastric pain, gastrointestinal (GI) bleeding, allergic reactions, nephrotoxicity and hepatotoxicity (with long-term use), tinnitus

Nursing Implications and Precautions:

- Use with caution in clients with asthma, bleeding or clotting disorders, unusual bruising, or peptic ulcers.
- Assess for aspirin hypersensitivity before administering drug.
- For clients concurrently taking anticoagulant medications, assess prothrombin time (PT) or international normalized ratio (INR) values before administering aspirin.
- Do not administer to children or teenagers with a fever because of the potential for Reye's syndrome.
- Administer with food and a full glass of water.
- For enteric-coated or extended release forms, advise clients to swallow the drug whole and not to crush, split, or chew the drug.
- Monitor for tinnitus and gradual hearing impairment.
- Advise client to limit or eliminate smoking and alcohol use because these increase the risk of GI bleeding.
- Advise the female client to immediately notify the prescriber of known or suspected pregnancy.

Side Effects: Bradycardia, hypotension, fatigue, dizziness, nausea, vomiting, tingling of the hands and feet, hyperglycemia

Nursing Implications and Precautions:

- Do not administer to clients with sinus bradycardia, heart block greater than first degree, cardiogenic shock, or overt heart failure.
- Monitor for impending cardiac failure (distended neck veins, edema, night cough, and dyspnea); discontinue drug and immediately notify prescriber.
- Advise client to not discontinue the drug abruptly because this may precipitate angina pain or myocardial infarction.
- Administer with caution to clients with diabetes, hyperthyroidism, or asthma.
- Advise client to move slowly from a lying to a standing position to prevent light-headedness.

Generic: atomoxetine (AT-oh-mox-ih-teen)

Brand: Strattera

Classification(s): ADHD agent; psychotherapeutic agent

Generic: atorvastatin (ah-torr-vah-STAH-tin)

Brand: Lipitor

Classification(s): Antilipemic; HMG-CoA reductase inhibitor; statin

Side Effects: Hepatotoxicity, sudden death (in clients with pre-existing structural cardiac abnormalities or other serious heart conditions), irritability, fatigue, nervousness, palpitations, anorexia, elevated blood pressure, mood or behavioral changes, dependence

Nursing Implications and Precautions:

- Monitor for signs of liver injury; discontinue drug and immediately notify prescriber.
- Assess the cardiovascular status (including family history) of the client prior to starting therapy.
- Monitor for suicidal ideation.
- Advise clients to swallow the drug whole and not to crush, split, or chew the capsules.
- Do not administer this drug to clients taking monoamine oxidase (MAO) inhibitors.

- In children, monitor growth and weight during therapy because this drug can suppress long-term growth.
- Advise parents of pediatric clients to immediately report aggression, hostility, mania, or other major behavioral problems.
- Use with caution in clients with cardiac disease, psychoses, or liver impairment.

Side Effects: Intestinal cramping, diarrhea, constipation, nasopharyngitis, arthralgia

Nursing Implications and Precautions:

- Monitor liver enzymes during therapy for possible hepatotoxicity.
- Do not administer to clients with active liver disease.
- Assess for myopathy (muscle pain and weakness).

- Instruct clients to not take with grapefruit juice.
- Instruct women of childbearing age to use effective birth control method (pregnancy Category X).
- Instruct lactating women not to breastfeed.

Generic: azithromycin (ah-ZITH-row-MYE-sin)

Brand: Zithromax

Classification(s): Antibiotic, macrolide

Generic: benazepril (ben-AY-zih-prill)

Brand: Lotensin

Classification(s): Antihypertensive; renin angiotensin system antagonist

Side Effects: Diarrhea, nausea, abdominal pain, angioedema (rare) and cholestatic jaundice (rare), allergic reactions

Nursing Implications and Precautions:

- Advise client to take drug for the entire length of time prescribed, even if symptoms of infection have resolved.

- Monitor for pseudomembranous colitis (severe diarrhea).

- Do not administer antacids within 2 hours of a dose of azithromycin.

- If client experiences an allergic reaction to the drug, monitor closely for several days because delayed symptoms may appear.

- Do not administer drug to clients with myasthenia gravis because symptoms may worsen.

- Assess for history of hypersensitivity to macrolides or other antibiotics.

Side Effects: Headache, cough, dizziness, orthostatic hypotension, angioedema, hyperkalemia, fetal death and injury

Nursing Implications and Precautions:

- Instruct women of childbearing age to use effective birth control method (pregnancy Category D).

- Advise the female client to immediately notify the prescriber of known or suspected pregnancy.

- Use with caution in clients with kidney or liver disease.

- Advise client to limit or eliminate alcohol use during therapy.

- Monitor blood pressure during therapy to evaluate drug effectiveness.

- Advise client to move slowly from a lying to a standing position to prevent light-headedness.

- Advise client to drink at least 6–8 glasses of water each day.

- Advise client to take drug for the entire length of time prescribed.

- Advise client not to use salt substitutes containing potassium, unless directed by the prescriber.

Generic: benzonatate (ben-ZOE-nah-tate)

Brand: Tessalon Perles

Classification(s): Antitussive; cough suppressant

Generic: bupropion (byoo-PRO-pee-on)

Brand: Wellbutrin, Zyban

Classification(s): Antidepressant

Side Effects: Hypersensitivity reactions, drowsiness, confusion, nasal stuffiness, headache, oropharyngeal anesthesia (if drug is chewed)

Nursing Implications and Precautions:

- Advise client to swallow the drug whole and not to suck on or chew the capsules because this can result in serious side effects.

- Assess client for history of allergy to procaine and similar anesthetics.

Side Effects: Suicidal ideation, anorexia, dry mouth, rash, tinnitus, sweating, nausea, tremor, migraine, seizures

Nursing Implications and Precautions:

- Monitor for worsening depression, unusual behavioral changes, and suicidal ideation.

- Advise clients taking this drug for smoking cessation to immediately report changes in mood, agitation, hostility, or delusions.

- Advise clients taking this drug for smoking cessation to not smoke or use any nicotine product because this may cause serious side effects.

- Advise client to continue taking the drug, even if feeling better.

- Use with caution in clients with seizure disorders or severe hepatic impairment.

- Advise client to move slowly from a lying to a standing position to prevent light-headedness.

- Do not administer this drug to clients taking monoamine oxidase (MAO) inhibitors.

- Advise client to not discontinue the drug abruptly.

- Advise client to limit or eliminate alcohol use during therapy because this increases the risk for seizures.

Generic: buspirone (byoo-SPY-rohn)

Brand: BuSpar

Classification(s): Antianxiety; anxiolytic

Generic: carisoprodol (kar-EE-soh-PROH-dole)

Brand: Soma

Classification(s): Skeletal muscle relaxant, central-acting

Side Effects: Dizziness, nausea, headache, nervousness, insomnia, light-headedness and excitement

Nursing Implications and Precautions:

- Do not administer this drug to clients taking monoamine oxidase (MAO) inhibitors.

- Advise client not to drive or operate hazardous machinery until the effects of the drug are known.

- Do not administer the drug with grapefruit juice.

- Advise client to not discontinue the drug abruptly.

- Advise client that the drug must be taken several weeks before the full effects of the drug are noticed.

- Advise client to limit or eliminate alcohol use during therapy because this increases drowsiness.

Side Effects: Dizziness, drowsiness, headache

Nursing Implications and Precautions:

- Advise client to limit or eliminate alcohol use during therapy because this increases drowsiness.

- Advise client not to drive or operate hazardous machinery until the effects of the drug are known.

- Use caution when administering other CNS depressants concurrently because this may cause additive sedation.

- Advise client to not discontinue the drug abruptly.

Generic: carvedilol (KAR-vih-DYE-loll)

Brand: Coreg

Classification(s): Antihypertensive; adrenergic blocker; alpha- and beta-adrenergic antagonist

Generic: cefdinir (SEF-dih-neer)

Brand: Omnicef

Classification(s): Antibiotic; third-generation cephalosporin

Side Effects: Left ventricular dysfunction (following myocardial infarction), bradycardia, hypotension, fatigue, dizziness, diarrhea, weight gain, hyperglycemia

Nursing Implications and Precautions:

- Do not administer to clients with severe bradycardia, heart block greater than first degree, cardiogenic shock, or decompensated heart failure.

- Monitor for worsening heart failure or fluid retention.

- Advise client to not discontinue the drug abruptly because this may precipitate angina pain or myocardial infarction.

- Monitor blood glucose levels in clients with diabetes.

- Administer with caution to clients with diabetes, severe hepatic impairment, hyperthyroidism, or asthma.

- Advise client to move slowly from a lying to a standing position to prevent light-headedness.

Side Effects: Diarrhea, nausea, vomiting, rash, allergic reactions

Nursing Implications and Precautions:

- Advise client to take drug for the entire length of time prescribed, even if symptoms of infection have resolved.

- Monitor for allergic reactions, including anaphylaxis.

- Monitor for pseudomembranous colitis (severe diarrhea).

- Monitor clients with mononucleosis carefully for skin rashes.

- Assess for history of hypersensitivity to cephalosporins or other antibiotics.

- Do not administer antacids or iron supplements within 2 hours of a dose of cefdinir.

Generic: celecoxib (sell-ah-COX-ib)

Brand: Celebrex

Classification(s): Analgesic, nonsteroidal anti-inflammatory (NSAID); antirheumatic; cyclooxygenase-2 (COX-2) inhibitor

Generic: cephalexin (sef-ah-LEX-in)

Brand: Keflex

Classification(s): Antibiotic, beta-lactam; first-generation cephalosporin

Side Effects: Abdominal pain, diarrhea, dyspepsia, flatulence, peripheral edema, accidental injury, dizziness, pharyngitis, rash, increased risk of thrombotic events, Stevens-Johnson syndrome, allergic reactions

Nursing Implications and Precautions:

- Monitor client during therapy for thrombotic events, myocardial infarction, and stroke.
- Use with caution in clients with a history of peptic ulcers or gastrointestinal bleeding, heart failure, or renal impairment.
- Monitor laboratory results for liver function; discontinue drug and notify prescriber if abnormal liver enzymes persist or worsen.

- Advise client to immediately report rash, blistering of the skin, or flu symptoms.
- Monitor for abnormal bleeding in clients taking warfarin because concurrent use may increase the risk of bleeding.
- Monitor blood pressure regularly during therapy.
- Assess for history of hypersensitivity to nonsteroidal anti-inflammatory drugs or sulfonamides.

Side Effects: Diarrhea, nausea, vomiting, rash, allergic reactions

Nursing Implications and Precautions:

- Advise client to take drug for the entire length of time prescribed, even if symptoms of infection have resolved.
- Monitor for allergic reactions, including anaphylaxis.
- Monitor for pseudomembranous colitis (severe diarrhea).
- Monitor clients with mononucleosis carefully for skin rashes.

- Assess for history of hypersensitivity to cephalosporins or other antibiotics.
- Do not administer antacids or iron supplements within 2 hours of a dose of cephalexin.
- Use caution when administering to clients with impaired renal function or with coagulation disorders.

Generic: **cetirizine** (sih-TEER-ah-zeen)

Brand: Zyrtec

Classification(s): Antihistamine, nonsedating; H_1-receptor antagonist

Generic: **chlorhexidine gluconate** (klor-HEX-ih-deen GLUE-kon-ayt)

Brand: Peridex, PerioGard

Classification(s): Antiseptic

Side Effects: Drowsiness, fatigue, dry mouth

Nursing Implications and Precautions:

- Advise client to avoid driving and other hazardous activities until the effects of the drug are known.

- Advise client to limit or eliminate alcohol use during therapy because this will increase drowsiness.

Side Effects: Increased staining of teeth and oral mucosa, increased calculus formation, altered taste perception, allergic reactions, stomatitis, gingivitis, dry mouth

Nursing Implications and Precautions:

- Advise client to brush and floss teeth daily and keep all appointments with dental professionals.

- Advise client that alterations in taste caused by the drug will diminish over time.

- Advise client to spit out the oral rinse after use and not to swallow the liquid.

Generic: chlorpheniramine (KLOR-fen-EER-ah-meen)

Brand: Chlor-Trimeton, many others

Classification(s): Antihistamine; H_1-receptor antagonist

Generic: ciprofloxacin (SEE-proh-FLOX-ah-sin)

Brand: Cipro, others

Classification(s): Antibiotic, quinolone

Side Effects: Drowsiness, headache, fatigue, dry mouth, thickening of bronchial secretions, excitement (especially in children), urinary retention

Nursing Implications and Precautions:

- Advise client to avoid driving and other hazardous activities until the effects of the drug are known.
- Advise client to limit or eliminate alcohol use during therapy because this will increase drowsiness.
- Use with caution in clients with emphysema, bronchitis, active gastric ulcers, glaucoma, or prostatic hyperplasia.
- Advise client to not crush, chew, or break extended-release forms of the drug.

Side Effects: Nausea, vomiting, headache, dizziness, tendinitis, tendon rupture, allergic reactions, Stevens-Johnson syndrome, photosensitivity, diarrhea

Nursing Implications and Precautions:

- Advise client to take drug for the entire length of time prescribed, even if symptoms of infection have resolved.
- Assess for history of hypersensitivity to fluoroquinolones or other antibiotics.
- Monitor for tendonitis or tendon rupture.
- Advise client to immediately report any unusual pain, inflammation, or swelling of joints, especially the Achilles tendon.
- Advise client to immediately report rash, blistering of the skin, or flu symptoms.
- Monitor for pseudomembranous colitis (severe diarrhea).
- Advise client to minimize exposure to direct sunlight and to wear protective clothing if exposed to the sun.
- Do not administer sucralfate or antacids containing magnesium or aluminum within 2 hours of a dose of ciprofloxacin.
- Advise client to not crush, chew, or break extended-release forms of the drug.
- Advise client to not take drug with dairy products or with calcium-fortified juice.

Generic: citalopram (sye-TAL-oh-pram)

Brand: Celexa

Classification(s): Antidepressant; selective serotonin reuptake inhibitor (SSRI)

Generic: clarithromycin (klah-RITH-row-MYE-sin)

Brand: Biaxin

Classification(s): Antibiotic, macrolide

Side Effects: Suicidal ideation, dry mouth, sedation, confusion, agitation, ejaculatory delay, drowsiness, abnormal bleeding, serotonin syndrome and neuroleptic malignant syndrome (rare)

Nursing Implications and Precautions:

- Do not administer to clients with suicidal ideation.

- Monitor for worsening depression and suicidal ideation.

- Advise client to avoid driving and other hazardous activities until the effects of the drug are known.

- Advise client to continue taking the drug, even if feeling better.

- Advise client that the drug must be taken several weeks before the full effects of the drug are noticed.

- Monitor for unusual bruising or bleeding.

- Advise client to not take aspirin or other drugs that affect coagulation unless directed by the prescriber.

- Do not administer this drug to clients taking monoamine oxidase (MAO) inhibitors.

- Advise client to limit or eliminate alcohol use during therapy because this may cause excessive drowsiness.

Side Effects: Diarrhea, nausea, abnormal taste, dyspepsia, abdominal pain, angioedema (rare), cholestatic jaundice (rare), and allergic reactions

Nursing Implications and Precautions:

- Advise client to take drug for the entire length of time prescribed, even if symptoms of infection have resolved.

- Monitor for pseudomembranous colitis (severe diarrhea).

- If client experiences an allergic reaction to the drug, monitor closely for several days because delayed symptoms may appear.

- Do not administer drug to clients with myasthenia gravis because symptoms may worsen.

- Advise client not to crush, chew, or split the extended release tablets.

Generic: clindamycin (KLIN-dah-MYE-sin)

Brand: Cleocin

Classification(s): Antibiotic, lincosamide

Generic: clonazepam (kloh-NAY-zih-pam)

Brand: Klonopin

Classification(s): Anticonvulsant; benzodiazepine

Side Effects: Diarrhea, nausea, abdominal pain, skin rash, jaundice

Nursing Implications and Precautions:

- Advise client to take drug for the entire length of time prescribed, even if symptoms of infection have resolved.
- Monitor for pseudomembranous colitis (severe diarrhea).
- Administer with caution in clients with history of gastrointestinal (GI) disease and atopic individuals.
- Monitor laboratory tests for hepatic and renal function.
- Do not administer this drug with erythromycin because they have antagonistic effects.

Side Effects: Dizziness, ataxia, drowsiness, sedation, confusion, dependence, blurred vision, seizures, birth defects (pregnancy Category D)

Nursing Implications and Precautions:

- Advise client to not discontinue the drug abruptly.
- Advise client to avoid driving and other hazardous activities until the effects of the drug are known.
- Do not administer to clients with suicidal ideation.
- Assess for signs of overdose or abuse (confusion, sedation, slurred speech, coma).
- Advise client to store drug in a safe place, away from children or those who may take the drug for recreational purposes.
- Advise the female client to immediately notify the prescriber of known or suspected pregnancy.
- Advise client to limit or eliminate alcohol use during therapy.
- Do not administer drug with grapefruit juice.
- Use caution when administering other CNS depressants concurrently with clonazepam due to the potential for excessive sedation.

Generic: clonidine (KLOH-nih-deen)

Brand: Catapress

Classification(s): Antihypertensive, central-acting; analgesic

Side Effects: Drowsiness, dizziness, constipation, palpitations, nervousness, agitation, nausea and vomiting

Nursing Implications and Precautions:

- Advise client to not discontinue the drug abruptly because this may cause a rapid rise in blood pressure.

- Continue administration of drug to within 4 hours of surgery, and resume as soon as possible following surgery.

- Advise client to avoid driving and other hazardous activities until the effects of the drug are known.

- Advise client to limit or eliminate alcohol use during therapy because this will increase drowsiness.

- Administer with caution in clients receiving digoxin, calcium channel blockers, or beta blockers because this increases the risk for arrhythmias.

- Advise client to move slowly from a lying to a standing position to prevent light-headedness.

Generic: clopidogrel (kloh-PID-oh-grel)

Brand: Plavix

Classification(s): Antithrombotic; antiplatelet; platelet aggregation inhibitor

Generic: clotrimazole (kloh-TRIM-ah-zole)

Brand: Gyne-Lotrimin, others

Classification(s): Antifungal, azole; antibiotic

Side Effects: Bleeding, bruising, thrombotic thrombocytopenia purpura (TTP)

Nursing Implications and Precautions:

- Monitor client carefully for unusual bleeding.
- Advise client to immediately report signs of bleeding, including nosebleeds and black/tarry stools.
- Do not administer to clients with active bleeding, including peptic ulcers and intracranial hemorrhage.
- Advise client to not discontinue the drug without consulting the health care provider because this increases the risk of bleeding.
- Use caution when using this drug with other anticoagulants such as aspirin or warfarin because this increases the risk for bleeding.
- Use with caution when concurrently administering drugs that inhibit the activity of CYPC219 enzyme (such as omeprazole) because this decreases the effectiveness of clopidogrel.

Side Effects: Local redness, stinging, blistering, peeling, edema, itching, or rash

Nursing Implications and Precautions:

- Advise client to take drug for the entire length of time prescribed, even if symptoms of infection have resolved.
- Advise client to avoid the use of occlusive dressings or wrappings around the infection site.
- Advise client to notify the prescriber if the area of infection does not improve after 4 weeks of therapy or if the infection worsens during therapy.
- For clients taking the lozenge form of the drug, monitor laboratory results of hepatic function during therapy.
- For clients taking the lozenge form of the drug, allow the lozenge to dissolve slowly in the mouth over 20–30 minutes.

Generic: codeine (KOH-deen)

Brand: Brontex, many others

Classification(s): Antitussive; narcotic (opiate agonist) analgesic

Generic: colchicine (COAL-chih-seen)

Brand: Colcrys

Classification(s): Antigout

Side Effects: Respiratory depression, light-headedness, sedation, nausea and vomiting, dysphoria, constipation, dependence

Nursing Implications and Precautions:

- Monitor carefully in clients with high potential for substance abuse.
- Do not administer to clients with head injury or high intracranial pressure.
- Monitor for interactions with other CNS depressants.
- Monitor for excessive sedation.
- Advise client to avoid driving and other hazardous activities until the effects of the drug are known.

- Advise client to limit or eliminate alcohol use during therapy because this may cause excessive drowsiness.
- Do not administer to clients with paralytic ileus, acute or severe asthma, or severe respiratory depression.
- Use with caution in clients with a history of drug abuse.

Side Effects: Diarrhea, pharyngolaryngeal pain, abdominal pain, nausea and vomiting, blood dyscrasias, rhabdomyolysis

Nursing Implications and Precautions:

- Advise client to store drug in a safe place, away from children.
- Monitor periodic laboratory tests for blood dyscrasias.
- Do not administer concurrently with strong CYP3A4 enzyme inhibitors (such as clarithromycin or cyclosporine).

- Monitor for muscle and joint pain, especially in clients receiving concurrent therapy with statin medications.
- Advise client to take drug exactly as prescribed and not to take it more frequently.

Generic: **cromolyn** (KROW-moe-lin)

Brand: Intal, Nasalcrom

Classification(s): Antiasthmatic; anti-inflammatory; mast cell stabilizer

Generic: **cyclobenzaprine** (SYE-kloh-BENZ-ah-preen)

Brand: Flexeril

Classification(s): Antispasmodic; skeletal muscle relaxant, central acting

Side Effects: Bronchospasm, cough, throat irritation, nasal congestion, local burning and stinging (intranasal form)

Nursing Implications and Precautions:

- If concurrently using a bronchodilator, administer the bronchodilator first and wait 5 minutes before using the cromolyn.

- Advise client that this drug should not be used to treat an acute asthma attack that has already begun.

- For asthma, administer Intal by oral inhalation; Nasalcrom is an intranasal form available over the counter for allergic rhinitis.

- Advise client that the drug must be taken several weeks before the full effects are noticed.

- Teach client the proper use of the face mask or mouthpiece device.

- Do not abruptly withdraw oral corticosteroids when switching to cromolyn.

Side Effects: Drowsiness, dry mouth, fatigue, dizziness, constipation, blurred vision

Nursing Implications and Precautions:

- Do not administer this drug to clients taking monoamine oxidase (MAO) inhibitors.

- Do not administer this drug to clients in the acute recovery phase of myocardial infarction, or to individuals with hyperthyroidism, arrhythmias, or congestive heart failure.

- Advise client that use with alcohol or other CNS depressants may cause excessive drowsiness.

- Administer with caution in clients with urinary retention, glaucoma, or hepatic impairment.

- Advise client to avoid driving and other hazardous activities until the effects of the drug are known.

- Administer with caution in older adult clients because they experience a higher incidence of CNS side effects such as confusion and hallucinations.

Generic: desloratidine (DEZ-lorr-AT-ah-deen)

Brand: Clarinex

Classification(s): Antihistamine, nonsedating; antiallergic; H_1-receptor antagonist

Generic: diazepam (die-AY-zih-pam)

Brand: Valium

Classification(s): Anticonvulsant; antianxiety; benzodiazepine; anxiolytic

Side Effects: Drowsiness, fatigue, dry mouth, headache

Nursing Implications and Precautions:

- Advise client to avoid driving and other hazardous activities until the effects of the drug are known.

- Advise client to limit or eliminate alcohol use during therapy because this may increase drowsiness.

Side Effects: Dizziness, ataxia, drowsiness, sedation, confusion, dependence, blurred vision, seizures, birth defects (pregnancy Category D)

Nursing Implications and Precautions:

- Advise client to not discontinue the drug abruptly.

- Advise client to avoid driving and other hazardous activities until the effects of the drug are known.

- Do not administer to clients with suicidal ideation.

- Assess for signs of overdose or abuse (confusion, sedation, slurred speech, coma).

- Advise client to store drug in a safe place, away from children or those who may take the drug for recreational purposes.

- Advise the female client to immediately notify the prescriber of known or suspected pregnancy.

- Advise client to limit or eliminate alcohol use during therapy because this will increase drowsiness.

- If administering by the intravenous route, use care to avoid extravasation, assess for phlebitis, and monitor for the possibility of apnea and /or cardiac arrest.

- Use caution when administering other CNS depressants concurrently with diazepam due to the potential for excessive sedation.

Generic: diclofenac (dye-KLOH-fen-ak)

Brand: Cataflam, others

Classification(s): Antipyretic; analgesic, nonsteroidal anti-inflammatory drug (NSAID)

Side Effects: Gastrointestinal (GI) ulceration or bleeding, abdominal pain, diarrhea, dyspepsia, peripheral edema, dizziness, rash, increased risk of thrombotic events, Stevens-Johnson syndrome, allergic reactions

Nursing Implications and Precautions:

- Monitor client during therapy for thrombotic events, myocardial infarction, and stroke.

- Do not administer drug for the treatment or peripoperative pain in the setting of coronary artery bypass graft surgery.

- Monitor client during therapy for GI bleeding.

- Administer with caution in clients with a history of peptic ulcers or gastrointestinal bleeding, heart failure, hypertension, or renal impairment.

- Monitor laboratory results for liver function; discontinue drug and notify prescriber if abnormal liver enzymes persist or worsen.

- Advise client to immediately report rash, blistering of the skin, or flu symptoms.

- Monitor for abnormal bleeding in clients taking warfarin because concurrent use may increase the risk of bleeding.

- Advise client to immediately report signs of hepatotoxicity (nausea, fatigue, jaundice, right upper quadrant pain).

- Monitor blood pressure regularly during therapy.

- Assess for history of hypersensitivity to nonsteroidal anti-inflammatory drugs.

Generic: dicyclomine (dye-SYE-kloh-meen)

Brand: Bentyl

Classification(s): GI antispasmodic; anticholinergic

Side Effects: Dry mouth, dizziness, blurred vision, nausea, drowsiness, weakness, nervousness

Nursing Implications and Precautions:

- Do not administer drug to clients with obstructive uropathy, obstructive disease of the gastrointestinal (GI) tract, severe ulcerative colitis, reflux esophagitis, glaucoma, or myasthenia gravis.

- Advise client to avoid high environmental temperatures or heavy exercise during therapy because heat stroke may occur.

- Advise client to avoid driving and other hazardous activities until the effects of the drug are known.

- Do not administer drug to infants less than 6 months of age.

- Advise client to limit or eliminate alcohol use during therapy because this may increase side effects from the drug.

Generic: digoxin (dig-OX-in)

Brand: Lanoxin, others

Classification(s): Antiarrhythmic; cardiac glycoside; inotropic

Side Effects: GI upset, anorexia, vision disturbances, confusion, headache, weakness, dizziness, gynecomastia, rash, heart block, arrhythmias

Nursing Implications and Precautions:

- Do not administer drug to clients with ventricular arrhythmias.

- Monitor for changes in vision, including blurred vision and changes in color vision.

- Monitor electrolytes frequently because drug toxicity is increased with hypokalemia, hypomagnesemia, and hypercalcemia.

- Monitor serum levels of digoxin.

- Monitor renal function during therapy; dose must be lowered in clients with renal impairment.

- Administer with caution to clients with serious cardiac disease, including sinus node disease, incomplete AV block, Wolff-Parkinson-White syndrome, restrictive cardiomyopathy, constrictive pericarditis, amyloid heart disease, acute cor pulmonale, idiopathic hypertrophic subaortic stenosis, or acute MI.

- If overdosage occurs, be prepared to administer digoxin immune fab (Digibind).

- Advise client to notify health care providers of all medications taken because digoxin interacts with multiple drugs.

Generic: diltiazem (dill-TYE-ah-zem)

Brand: Cardizem, others

Classification(s): Antihypertensive; antianginal; antiarrhythmic; calcium channel blocking agent

Generic: diphenhydramine (DYE-fen-HYE-drah-meen)

Brand: Benadryl

Classification(s): Antihistamine; sedative-hypnotic; antiparkinson; antidyskinetic; nonnarcotic antitussive; centrally acting cholinergic antagonist; H_1-receptor antagonist

Side Effects: Flushing, hypotension, headache, dizziness, peripheral edema, reflex tachycardia

Nursing Implications and Precautions:

- Assess for swelling of hands, feet, and ankles.
- Use with caution in clients with bradycardia, sick sinus syndrome, heart failure, or hepatic impairment.
- Monitor blood pressure periodically to ensure drug effectiveness.
- Advise client to continue taking the drug, even if symptoms resolve.
- Advise client to limit or eliminate alcohol use during therapy.
- Advise client to move slowly from a lying to a standing position to prevent light-headedness.
- Monitor client carefully when beginning therapy or changing doses because this may worsen angina pain or cause a myocardial infarction.
- Advise clients taking extended-release forms to swallow the drug whole and not to crush, split, or chew the capsules.

Side Effects: Drowsiness, anticholinergic effects (dry mouth, dizziness, blurred vision, nausea), excitability in children

Nursing Implications and Precautions:

- Do not administer this drug to neonates or premature infants.
- Advise client to not use multiple products concurrently that contain this drug (cold, allergy, sinus, topical, etc.).
- Administer with caution to clients with asthma, glaucoma, hyperthyroidism, hypertension, cardiovascular disease, or gastrointestinal (GI) or urinary obstruction.
- Advise client to avoid driving and other hazardous activities until the effects of the drug are known.
- Advise client to limit or eliminate alcohol use during therapy because this may cause excessive drowsiness.
- Monitor older adult clients carefully because side effects are more pronounced in this population.

Generic: divalproex sodium (DYE-val-PROH-ex)

Brand: Depakote

Classification(s): Anticonvulsant; gamma-aminobutyric acid (GABA) inhibitor

Side Effects: Dizziness, headache, GI upset, asthenia, tremor, drowsiness, endocrine effects, blood dyscrasias, thrombocytopenia, hepatotoxicity, acute pancreatitis, birth defects (pregnancy Category D), hyperammonemia

Nursing Implications and Precautions:

- Assess hepatic function prior to therapy and do not administer drug to clients with severe hepatic impairment or urea cycle disorders.

- Monitor liver enzyme tests at frequent intervals during therapy for possible hepatotoxicity.

- Monitor for suicidal ideation.

- Advise client to not discontinue the drug abruptly because seizures may occur.

- Administer with caution to clients on multiple anticonvulsants, those with congenital metabolic disorders, severe seizure disorders accompanied by mental retardation, or organic brain disease and children under age 2.

- Monitor for pancreatitis (abdominal pain, nausea, vomiting, and anorexia).

- Advise the female client to immediately notify the prescriber of known or suspected pregnancy.

- Monitor for hyperammonemia (lethargy, vomiting, or changes in mental status).

- Monitor for bleeding and laboratory values of platelets.

Generic: donepezil (doh-NEP-ih-zil)

Brand: Aricept

Classification(s): Antidementia; Alzheimer's agent; central-acting cholinergic; cholinesterase inhibitor

Generic: doxazosin (dox-AY-zoh-sin)

Brand: Cardura

Classification(s): Antihypertensive; alpha-adrenergic antagonist

Side Effects: Nausea, vomiting, insomnia, muscle cramps, fatigue, anorexia, weight loss

Nursing Implications and Precautions:

- Administer with caution to clients with cardiac conduction conditions, peptic ulcer, digestive or urinary obstruction, seizures, asthma, or chronic obstructive pulmonary disease.
- Monitor for GI bleeding.
- Monitor calorie intake and body weight during therapy.

- Advise client to avoid driving and other hazardous activities until the effects of the drug are known.
- For the orally disintegrating tablet (ODT), advise client to allow the tablet to dissolve slowly in the mouth without chewing or swallowing the tablet whole.

Side Effects: Syncope (first-dose effect), dizziness, drowsiness, fatigue, edema, dyspnea, blurred vision, orthostatic hypotension, arrhythmia, priapism (rare)

Nursing Implications and Precautions:

- Monitor blood pressure during therapy to evaluate drug effectiveness.
- Advise client to move slowly from a lying to a standing position to prevent light-headedness.
- Monitor client carefully for hypotension following the first dose and when dosages are increased.
- Advise client to take drug at bedtime to avoid drowsiness or dizziness.

- Advise the male client to immediately report a penis erection that is painful and lasts 4 hours or longer because this may result in permanent damage to erectile tissue.
- Administer with caution to clients with hepatic impairment.
- Assess for prostate cancer prior to treatment because this drug is contraindicated in these clients.
- Advise clients taking extended-release forms to swallow the drug whole and not to crush, split, or chew the tablets.

Generic: doxycycline (DOX-ee-SYE-kleen)

Brand: Doryx, others

Classification(s): Antibiotic, tetracycline

Side Effects: Photosensitivity, GI upset (anorexia, nausea vomiting), rash, blood dyscrasias, fetal toxicity (pregnancy Category D), allergic reaction, teeth discoloration in children

Nursing Implications and Precautions:

- Advise client to take drug for the entire length of time prescribed, even if symptoms of infection have resolved.

- Do not administer this drug to children under age 8 years because permanent teeth discoloration may occur.

- Monitor for pseudomembranous colitis (severe diarrhea).

- Advise client to minimize exposure to direct sunlight and to wear protective clothing if exposed to the sun.

- Advise the female client to immediately notify the prescriber of known or suspected pregnancy.

- Monitor blood laboratory values during therapy.

- Do not administer zinc, iron, calcium, magnesium, or aluminum within 2 hours of a dose of doxycycline.

- Advise female clients taking oral contraceptives to use an additional method of birth control because doxycycline renders these drugs less effective.

Generic: duloxetine (du-LOX-ih-teen)

Brand: Cymbalta

Classification(s): Antidepressant; antianxiety; neuropathic pain reliever; serotonin norepinephrine reuptake inhibitor (SNRI)

Side Effects: Suicidal ideation, decreased appetite, dry mouth, drowsiness, sweating, nausea, hepatotoxicity, abnormal bleeding, serotonin syndrome (rare) and neuroleptic malignant syndrome (rare)

Nursing Implications and Precautions:

- Monitor for worsening depression, unusual behavioral changes, and suicidal ideation.
- Advise client to continue taking the drug, even if feeling better.
- Monitor liver enzyme tests for possible hepatotoxicity.
- Do not administer this drug to clients taking monoamine oxidase (MAO) inhibitors.
- Advise client to not discontinue the drug abruptly.
- Use with caution in clients with seizure disorders, severe kidney disease, hepatic impairment or uncontrolled narrow-angle glaucoma.
- Advise client to limit or eliminate alcohol use during therapy because this increases the risk for liver injury.
- Monitor for abnormal bruising and bleeding.
- Advise client to not take aspirin or other drugs that affect coagulation unless directed by the prescriber.
- Monitor blood pressure during therapy.

Generic: enalapril (ee-NALL-ah-prill)

Brand: Vasotec

Classification(s): Antihypertensive; angiotensin-converting enzyme (ACE) inhibitor

Generic: epinephrine (EP-ee-NEF-rin)

Brand: EpiPen, others

Classification(s): Antianaphylactic; vasopressor; alpha- and beta-adrenergic agonist; cardiac stimulant

Side Effects: Headache, cough, dizziness, orthostatic hypotension, angioedema, fetal death and injury

Nursing Implications and Precautions:

- Instruct women of childbearing age to use effective birth control method (pregnancy Category D).
- Advise the female client to immediately notify the prescriber of known or suspected pregnancy.
- Use with caution in clients with kidney or liver disease.
- Advise client to limit or eliminate alcohol use during therapy.
- Monitor blood pressure during therapy to evaluate drug effectiveness.
- Advise client to move slowly from a lying to a standing position to prevent light-headedness.
- Advise client to drink at least 6–8 glasses of water each day.
- Advise client to take drug for the entire length of time prescribed.
- Advise client not to use salt substitutes containing potassium, unless directed by the prescriber.

Side Effects: Anxiety, headache, fear, palpitations, arrhythmias, hypertension

Nursing Implications and Precautions:

- Do not administer to clients with angle closure glaucoma or nonanaphylactic shock.
- Administer with caution to clients with diabetes, thyroid disorders, arrhythmias, hypertension, or severe cardiac disease.
- Monitor blood pressure during therapy.
- Assess for extravasation because this drug may cause necrosis of tissue at injection sites.
- Protect drug from exposure to light and discard if the color appears pink or if a precipitate is present.

Generic: epoetin alfa (eh-POH-eh-tin AL-fah)

Brand: Epogen, others

Classification(s): Antianemic; human erythropoietin; hematopoietic growth factor

Generic: erythromycin (eh-RITH-row-MY-sin)

Brand: E-mycin

Classification(s): Antibiotic, macrolide

Side Effects: Iron deficiency, hypertension, headache, arthralgia, GI disturbances, edema, paresthesia, pyrexia, respiratory congestion, seizures; increased risk of death, thrombotic events, and tumor progression

Nursing Implications and Precautions:

- Monitor hemoglobin regularly; withhold dose if hemoglobin exceeds 12 g/dL.
- Do not administer to clients with uncontrolled hypertension.
- Administer with caution in clients with chronic renal failure.
- Monitor renal function regularly during therapy.
- Monitor serum iron, ferritin, and transferrin saturation before and during therapy; all clients will require iron supplementation.
- Monitor for thrombotic events during therapy.
- Monitor blood pressure regularly during therapy.
- Do not shake the vial because this may inactivate the drug.

Side Effects: Diarrhea, nausea, anorexia, dyspepsia, abdominal pain, angioedema (rare), ototoxicity, hepatotoxicity, allergic reactions

Nursing Implications and Precautions:

- Advise client to take drug for the entire length of time prescribed, even if symptoms of infection have resolved.
- Monitor for pseudomembranous colitis (severe diarrhea).
- Monitor laboratory tests of hepatic function for hepatotoxicity.
- If client experiences an allergic reaction to the drug, monitor closely for several days because delayed symptoms may appear.
- Do not administer drug to clients with myasthenia gravis because symptoms may worsen.
- Advise client not to crush, chew, or split extended release tablets or capsules.
- Monitor for hearing changes during therapy.

Generic: escitalopram (ESS-sye-TAH-loh-pram)

Brand: Lexapro

Classification(s): Antidepressant; selective serotonin reuptake inhibitor (SSRI)

Side Effects: Suicidal ideation, insomnia, sedation, fatigue, agitation, sexual disorders, drowsiness, abnormal bleeding, sweating, serotonin syndrome and neuroleptic malignant syndrome (rare)

Nursing Implications and Precautions:

- Do not administer to clients with suicidal ideation.
- Monitor for worsening depression and suicidal ideation.
- Advise client to avoid driving and other hazardous activities until the effects of the drug are known.
- Advise client to continue taking the drug, even if feeling better.
- Advise client that the drug must be taken several weeks before the full effects of the drug are noticed.
- Monitor for unusual bruising or bleeding.

- Advise client to not take aspirin or other drugs that affect coagulation unless directed by the prescriber.
- Do not administer this drug to clients taking monoamine oxidase (MAO) inhibitors.
- Advise client to limit or eliminate alcohol use during therapy because this may cause excessive drowsiness.
- Advise client to report changes in sexual performance, including ejaculatory delay, decreased libido, and anorgasmia.

Generic: esomeprazole (EE-soh-MEP-rah-zole)

Brand: Nexium

Classification(s): Antiulcer; proton pump inhibitor

Side Effects: Headache, diarrhea, abdominal pain, nausea, flatulence, constipation, dry mouth

Nursing Implications and Precautions:

• Administer with caution with drugs for which gastric pH affects bioavailability (such as ketoconazole, iron salts, and digoxin).

• Administer drug at least 1 hour before a meal.

• Advise clients taking extended-release forms to swallow the drug whole and not to crush, split, or chew the capsules.

• Advise client to continue taking the drug for the entire length of time prescribed, even if feeling better.

• Advise client to notify the prescriber if symptoms have not resolved following 4–8 weeks of therapy.

Generic: estradiol (ESS-trah-DYE-oll)

Brand: Estrace

Classification(s): Estrogen replacement

Side Effects: Irregular vaginal bleeding, amenorrhea, headache, hypertension, edema, hypercalcemia, gallbladder disease, thromboembolic disease (myocardial infarction, stroke, and pulmonary embolism), birth defects (pregnancy Category X), endometrial cancer

Nursing Implications and Precautions:

- Do not administer to clients with estrogen-dependent neoplasms, thrombophlebitis, thromboembolic disorders, or undiagnosed abnormal genital bleeding.

- Do not administer to pregnant clients; advise the female client to immediately notify the prescriber of known or suspected pregnancy.

- Administer with caution to clients with asthma, hepatic impairment, edema, or familial hyperlipoproteinemia.

- Monitor for liver impairment and discontinue drug if jaundice occurs.

- Monitor for recurring abnormal vaginal bleeding during therapy because this may indicate undiagnosed uterine cancer.

- Advise clients to implement lifestyle changes that reduce the risk for thromboembolic side effects (such as weight management and tobacco cessation).

- Monitor blood pressure at frequent intervals during therapy.

Generic: estrogens, conjugated (ESS-troh-jens, KON-ju-GAY-tid)

Brand: Premarin

Classification(s): Female hormone replacement therapy (HRT); estrogens

Side Effects: Irregular vaginal bleeding, amenorrhea, headache, hypertension, edema, hypercalcemia, gallbladder disease, thromboembolic disease (myocardial infarction, stroke, and pulmonary embolism), birth defects (pregnancy Category X), endometrial cancer

Nursing Implications and Precautions:

- Do not administer to clients with estrogen-dependent neoplasms, thrombophlebitis, thromboembolic disorders, or undiagnosed abnormal genital bleeding.

- Do not administer to pregnant clients; advise the female client to immediately notify the prescriber of known or suspected pregnancy.

- Administer with caution to clients with asthma, hepatic impairment, or edema.

- Monitor for liver impairment and discontinue drug if jaundice occurs.

- Monitor for recurring abnormal vaginal bleeding during therapy because this may indicate undiagnosed uterine cancer.

- Advise clients to implement lifestyle changes that reduce the risk for thromboembolic side effects (such as weight management and tobacco cessation).

- Monitor blood pressure at frequent intervals during therapy.

Generic: eszopiclone (ess-ZOP-ih-klone)

Brand: Lunesta

Classification(s): Sedative-hypnotic

Side Effects: Unpleasant taste, drowsiness, behavioral changes, complex sleep-related behaviors (such as having sex, driving, or eating while not fully awake), symptoms of the common cold, anaphylaxis

Nursing Implications and Precautions:

- Advise client to limit or eliminate alcohol use during therapy because this increases the side effects of the drug.

- Advise client to take drug exactly as prescribed and not to take higher amounts.

- Monitor for behavioral changes such as aggressiveness, agitation, hallucinations, or bizarre sleep behaviors.

- Advise client to take the drug immediately prior to expected sleep.

- Advise client to avoid driving and other hazardous activities until the effects of the drug are known.

- Administer with caution in clients with depression, suicidal ideation, or history of substance abuse.

- Advise client to notify the prescriber if insomnia does not improve after 7–10 days of therapy.

- Advise client to store drug in a safe place, away from children.

Generic: ethinyl estradiol and **norgestimate** (ETH-in-ill es-trah-DYE-oll/nor-JESS-tim-ate)

Brand: Ortho Tri-Cyclen, others

Classification(s): Estrogen; female hormone replacement therapy (HRT)

Side Effects: Hypertension, nausea, vomiting, irregular vaginal bleeding, amenorrhea, edema, headache, gallbladder disease, depression, thromboembolic disease (myocardial infarction, stroke, and pulmonary embolism)

Nursing Implications and Precautions:

- Do not administer to clients with known or suspected breast cancer, estrogen-dependent neoplasms, thrombophlebitis, thromboembolic disorders, valvular heart disease, headaches with focal neurological symptoms, jaundice with prior oral contraceptive use, known or suspected pregnancy or undiagnosed abnormal genital bleeding.

- Administer with caution to smokers over age 35 and clients with uncontrolled hypertension.

- Advise the female client to immediately notify the prescriber of known or suspected pregnancy.

- Monitor for liver impairment and discontinue drug if jaundice occurs.

- Advise smoking clients to discontinue tobacco use during therapy.

- Monitor blood pressure at frequent intervals during therapy.

- Assess for history of depression and discontinue drug if depression worsens during therapy.

- Monitor for recurring abnormal vaginal bleeding during therapy because this may indicate undiagnosed uterine cancer.

Generic: etodolac (EE-tow-DOH-lak)

Brand: Lodine

Classification(s): Analgesic, nonsteroidal anti-inflammatory agent (NSAID); disease-modifying antirheumatic drug (DMARD)

Side Effects: Gastrointestinal (GI) ulceration or bleeding, abdominal pain, diarrhea, dyspepsia, peripheral edema, dizziness, rash, increased risk of thrombotic events, Stevens-Johnson syndrome, allergic reactions

Nursing Implications and Precautions:

- Monitor client during therapy for thrombotic events, myocardial infarction, and stroke.

- Do not administer drug for the treatment or peripoperative pain in the setting of coronary artery bypass graft surgery.

- Monitor client during therapy for GI bleeding.

- Administer with caution in clients with a history of peptic ulcers or gastrointestinal bleeding, heart failure, hypertension, or renal impairment.

- Monitor laboratory results for liver function; discontinue drug and notify prescriber if abnormal liver enzymes persist or worsen.

- Advise client to immediately report rash, blistering of the skin, or flu symptoms.

- Monitor for abnormal bleeding in clients taking warfarin because concurrent use may increase the risk of bleeding.

- Advise client to immediately report signs of hepatotoxicity (nausea, fatigue, jaundice, right upper quadrant pain).

- Monitor blood pressure regularly during therapy.

- Assess for history of hypersensitivity to nonsteroidal anti-inflammatory drugs.

Generic: ezetimibe (eh-ZET-ih-mibe)

Brand: Zetia

Classification(s): Antilipemic; cholesterol absorption inhibitor

Generic: famotidine (fam-OH-ti-deen)

Brand: Pepcid

Classification(s): Antiulcer; antisecretory (H_2-receptor antagonist)

Side Effects: Upper respiratory tract infection, extremity pain, arthralgia, diarrhea, myopathy/rhabdomyolysis (if used with a statin)

Nursing Implications and Precautions:

- Do not administer drug with active liver disease or unexplained persistent elevations in serum transaminases.
- Administer with caution to clients with hepatic insufficiency.
- If administered concurrently with a statin, monitor liver function.

- Advise client to immediately report unexplained skeletal muscle pain or weakness.
- If administered with fibrates, monitor laboratory tests for gallbladder function.
- If administered with other cholesterol medications, ezetimibe should be taken at least 2 hours before cholestyramine, colestipol, or colesevelam.

Side Effects: Headache, dizziness, constipation, diarrhea

Nursing Implications and Precautions:

- Administer with caution to clients with moderate to severe renal impairment. Advise client to notify the prescriber if symptoms have not resolved in 4–6 weeks.

- Advise client to take drug for the entire length of time prescribed, even if symptoms have resolved.
- Administer drug 15–60 minutes before eating food or drinks that cause heartburn.

Generic: felodipine (feh-LOW-dih-peen)

Brand: Plendil

Classification(s): Antihypertensive; calcium channel blocker

Side Effects: Flushing, hypotension, headache, dizziness, peripheral edema, reflex tachycardia

Nursing Implications and Precautions:

- Assess for swelling of hands, feet, and ankles.
- Use with caution in clients with heart failure or hepatic impairment.
- Monitor blood pressure periodically to ensure drug effectiveness.
- Advise client to continue taking the drug, even if symptoms resolve.
- Do not administer the drug with grapefruit juice.

- Advise client to limit or eliminate alcohol use during therapy.
- Advise client to move slowly from a lying to a standing position to prevent light-headedness.
- Monitor client carefully when beginning therapy or changing doses because this may worsen angina pain or cause a myocardial infarction.

Generic: fenofibrate (FEN-oh-FYE-brate)

Brand: Tricor

Classification(s): Antilipemic; fibrate

Side Effects: Increased hepatic enzymes, myopathy, cholelithiasis, pancreatitis, increased blood urea nitrogen (BUN) or creatinine, rash

Nursing Implications and Precautions:

- Do not administer to clients with hepatic dysfunction, primary biliary cirrhosis, severe renal impairment, or gallbladder disease.

- Administer with caution to clients with renal impairment.

- Monitor complete blood counts (CBCs) for first year of therapy.

- Monitor liver function and discontinue drug if persistent elevated hepatic enzymes, myopathy, or gallstones occur.

- Administer with caution with statins because this increases the risk for side effects.

- If administered concurrently with anticoagulants, regularly monitor prothrombin/INR values.

- Monitor for the development of gallbladder disease during therapy.

- Monitor serum lipid levels during therapy to assess drug effectiveness.

- Advise client to immediately report unexplained skeletal muscle pain or weakness.

Generic: fentanyl transdermal (FEN-tah-nill)

Brand: Duragesic

Classification(s): Narcotic analgesic (opiate agonist)

Side Effects: Respiratory depression, light-headedness, sedation, nausea and vomiting, dysphoria, constipation, dependence

Nursing Implications and Precautions:

- Advise client to store drug in a safe place, away from children or those who may take the drug for recreational purposes.

- Monitor carefully in clients with high potential for substance abuse.

- Do not administer to clients with head injury or high intracranial pressure.

- Monitor for interactions with other CNS depressants.

- Monitor for excessive sedation.

- Advise client to avoid driving and other hazardous activities until the effects of the drug are known.

- Advise client to limit or eliminate alcohol use during therapy because this may cause excessive drowsiness.

- Monitor continuously for respiratory depression, which can be life threatening.

- Do not administer to clients unless they are opioid tolerant.

- Administer with caution when concurrently administering drugs that inhibit the activity of CYP3A4 enzyme (such as ritonavir, ketoconazole, erythromycin, or diltiazem) because this prolongs the adverse effects of fentanyl.

- Advise client to not use a patch if the seal is broken, cut, or damaged.

- Advise client to avoid all heat sources at the patch application site, such as heating pads, hot tubs, tanning lamps, or extended direct sunlight.

- Advise client to never use more patches per day than prescribed.

Generic: ferrous sulfate (FAIR-uss SULL-fate)

Brand: Feosol, Feratab, Fer-In-Sol, SlowFe

Classification(s): Antianemic; iron supplement

Generic: fexofenadine (FEX-oh-FEN-ah-deen)

Brand: Allegra

Classification(s): Nonsedating antihistamine; H_1-receptor antagonist

Side Effects: Nausea, abdominal pain, nausea, constipation, diarrhea, darkened or black stools, tooth discoloration (liquid forms)

Nursing Implications and Precautions:

- Do not administer to clients with hemochromatosis or hemosiderosis.

- Monitor hemoglobin, hematocrit, and reticulocyte count periodically to determine drug effectiveness.

- Administer with caution concurrently with tetracycline because iron inhibits its absorption.

- Administer on an empty stomach (if tolerated) 1 hour before or 2 hours after a meal. If stomach discomfort occurs, administer immediately after a meal.

- Advise client to keep medicine in a secure place because iron is toxic to children.

- Advise client not to take this drug at the same time as antacids or calcium supplements.

- To prevent staining of teeth, advise client to drink the liquid iron through a straw on the back of the tongue and rinse the mouth thoroughly after the dose is completed.

Side Effects: Headache, nausea, vomiting, increased incidence of viral infections, dry mouth

Nursing Implications and Precautions:

- Advise client to avoid driving and other hazardous activities until the effects of the drug are known.

- Advise client to limit or eliminate alcohol use during therapy because this will increase drowsiness.

- Do not administer concurrently with antacids containing magnesium or aluminum.

- For the orally disintegrating tablet (ODT), advise client to take the medication on an empty stomach and allow the tablet to dissolve slowly in the mouth without chewing or swallowing the tablet whole.

Generic: filgrastim (fill-GRASS-tim)

Brand: Neupogen

Classification(s): Antineutropenic; granulocyte colony-stimulating factor (G-CSF); hematopoietic growth factor

Generic: finasteride (fye-NASS-ter-ide)

Brand: Proscar

Classification(s): Antiandrogen; 5-alpha reductase inhibitor

Side Effects: Bone pain, petechiae, splenomegaly, epistaxis, transfusion reactions, allergic reactions, nausea/vomiting

Nursing Implications and Precautions:

- Do not administer to clients with hypersensitivity to *E. coli* products.

- Administer with caution to clients with pre-existing cardiac disease, or hyperplastic skin conditions, or sickle cell disease.

- Monitor complete blood count with differential before and regularly during therapy.

- Discontinue drug if postnadir absolute neutrophil count (ANC) reaches 10,000/mm^3 for clients receiving myelosuppressive chemotherapy.

- Monitor for splenomegaly/ splenic rupture.

- Monitor for adult respiratory distress syndrome (ARDS) and suspend therapy if this occurs.

- Monitor for serious allergic reactions.

- Advise client to take drug exactly as prescribed and not to take it more frequently.

- Teach client proper method of preparing and self-injecting the drug.

- Advise client not to shake the medication vial because this can inactivate the drug.

- Advise client to use disposable needles only once, and to dispose of them properly.

Side Effects: Impotence, diminished libido, decreased ejaculate volume, breast enlargement, birth defects (pregnancy Category X)

Nursing Implications and Precautions:

- Do not administer to pregnant women or those who could potentially be pregnant.

- Administer with caution to clients with hepatic impairment.

- Monitor prostate-specific antigen (PSA) levels during therapy.

- Monitor for prostate cancer and obstructive uropathy.

- Assess for prostate cancer prior to starting therapy.

- Advise pregnant women not to handle crushed or broken tablets because the drug may be absorbed through the skin.

Generic: fluconazole (floo-KOH-nah-zole)

Brand: Diflucan

Classification(s): Azole antifungal

Side Effects: Nausea, headache, rash, vomiting, diarrhea, abdominal pain, hepatotoxicity (rare), exfoliative dermatitis (rare)

Nursing Implications and Precautions:

- Do not administer concurrently with cisapride.
- Administer with caution to clients with history of arrythmias and with medications known to promote arrythmias.
- Monitor liver function and discontinue drug if liver disease worsens.
- Monitor for skin rash and discontinue drug if progressively worsening rash develops.
- Monitor for hypoglycemia in clients concurrently taking oral hypoglycemic drugs.
- Monitor prothrombin time regularly in clients concurrently taking warfarin (Coumadin).
- Advise client to take drug for the entire length of time prescribed, even if symptoms of infection have resolved.

Generic: fluoxetine (flu-OX-ah-teen)

Brand: Prozac, others

Classification(s): Antidepressant; selective serotonin reuptake inhibitor (SSRI)

Side Effects: Suicidal ideation, insomnia, weight changes (either gain or loss), nausea, vomiting, sexual disorders, drowsiness, abnormal bleeding, sweating, serotonin syndrome and neuroleptic malignant syndrome (rare)

Nursing Implications and Precautions:

- Do not administer to clients with suicidal ideation.
- Monitor for worsening depression and suicidal ideation.
- Advise client to avoid driving and other hazardous activities until the effects of the drug are known.
- Advise client to continue taking the drug, even if feeling better.
- Advise client that the drug must be taken several weeks before the full effects of the drug are noticed.
- Monitor for unusual bruising or bleeding.
- Advise client to not take aspirin or other drugs that affect coagulation unless directed by the prescriber.
- Do not administer this drug to clients taking monoamine oxidase (MAO) inhibitors.
- Advise client to limit or eliminate alcohol use during therapy because this may cause excessive drowsiness.
- Advise client to report changes in sexual performance, including ejaculatory delay, decreased libido, and anorgasmia.
- Monitor for weight gain or loss during therapy.

Generic: fluticasone (floo-TIK-ah-sone)

Brand: Flovent HFA, Flonase

Classification(s): Corticosteroid

Generic: folic acid (FOH-lik AH-sid)

Brand: Folvite

Classification(s): Vitamin B_9 supplement

Side Effects: Headache, pharyngitis, epistaxis, nasal burning, asthma symptoms, GI upset, cough

Nursing Implications and Precautions:

- Advise client to take drug for the entire length of time prescribed, even if symptoms have resolved.

- Monitor for adrenal insufficiency if client is concurrently receiving other systemic or topical corticosteroids.

- Advise client to take drug exactly as prescribed and not to take it more frequently.

- Monitor for localized *Candida* infection and other nasal mucosal changes.

- Administer with caution to clients with tuberculosis or other infections such as chickenpox, measles, or ocular herpes simplex.

- If exposed to measles or chickenpox, consider anti-infective prophylactic therapy. Monitor for growth reduction in children.

- Administer with caution to clients concurrently receiving strong CYP450 3A4 inhibitors (such as ketoconazole and ritonavir).

Side Effects: Allergic sensitization (erythema, skin rash, itching, malaise, bronchospasm)

Nursing Implications and Precautions:

- Administer the injectable form if disease is severe or gastrointestinal (GI) absorption is impaired.

- Assess client to rule out or treat vitamin B_{12} deficiency prior to treatment.

- Advise client not to concurrently take multivitamins containing folic acid unless approved by the prescriber.

Generic: furosemide (fyur-OH-suh-mide)

Brand: Lasix

Classification(s): Loop diuretic; antihypertensive; electrolytic and water balance agent

Generic: gabapentin (GAB-ah-PEN-tin)

Brand: Neurontin

Classification(s): Anticonvulsant; GABA analog

Side Effects: Fluid or electrolyte imbalance, GI upset, dizziness, orthostatic hypotension, hyperglycemia, jaundice, hyperuricemia, rash, ototoxicity, renal calcification in premature infants

Nursing Implications and Precautions:

- Do not administer to clients with anuria, hepatic coma, or untreated electrolyte depletion.
- Administer with caution to clients with renal or hepatic dysfunction, diabetes, gout, lupus, or sulfonamide sensitivity.
- Monitor blood pressure, serum electrolytes, and urinary output.
- Administer potassium supplements as prescribed.
- Monitor kidney function during therapy and discontinue if progressive renal impairment occurs.
- Monitor for hearing loss during therapy.
- Administer with caution with other ototoxic drugs such as aminoglycosides or ethacrynic acid.
- Monitor periodic blood glucose levels in clients with diabetes.

Side Effects: Somnolence, dizziness, ataxia, fatigue, nystagmus, visual disturbances, tremor, nausea/vomiting, dysarthria, confusion, dry mouth

Nursing Implications and Precautions:

- Do not administer to clients with serious renal impairment.
- Do not administer to clients with suicidal ideation.
- Monitor for suicidal ideation.
- Advise client to not discontinue the drug abruptly because this may cause seizures.
- Advise client to limit or eliminate alcohol use during therapy because this increases drowsiness.
- Administer at least 2 hours after antacids.
- In children ages 3–12 years, monitor for emotional lability, hostility, changes in school performance, and hyperactivity.
- Advise client to avoid driving and other hazardous activities until the effects of the drug are known.
- Advise client to continue taking the drug, even if feeling better.

Generic: **gemfibrozil** (jem-FYE-bro-zill)

Brand: Lopid

Classification(s): Antilipemic; fibrate

Side Effects: Dyspepsia, abdominal pain, acute appendicitis, atrial fibrillation, gallbladder disease, blurred vision, paresthesias, altered taste, dizziness, headache, impotence, myopathy, arthralgia, abnormal liver function tests, rash

Nursing Implications and Precautions:

- Do not administer to clients with hepatic dysfunction, primary biliary cirrhosis, or gallbladder disease.

- Monitor serum lipid levels during therapy to assess drug effectiveness.

- Monitor liver function and discontinue drug if persistent elevated hepatic enzymes, myopathy, or gallstones occur.

- Monitor complete blood counts (CBCs) for first year of therapy.

- Advise client to immediately report unexplained skeletal muscle pain or weakness.

- If administered concurrently with anticoagulants, regularly monitor prothrombin/INR values.

- Administer with caution with statins because this increases the risk for side effects.

- Monitor for the development of gallbladder disease during therapy.

- Administer with caution to clients with renal impairment.

Generic: gentamicin: jen-tuh-MYE-sin

Brand: Garamycin

Classification(s): Aminoglycoside antibiotic

Side Effects: Nephrotoxicity, ototoxicity, respiratory depression, lethargy, confusion, visual disturbances, blood dyscrasias, birth defects (pregnancy Category D)

Nursing Implications and Precautions:

- Monitor renal function regularly for nephrotoxicity.
- Monitor for hearing and balance impairment during therapy.
- Monitor serum drug levels: Avoid peak serum levels above 12 micrograms/mL (when dosed at conventional intervals) and trough levels above 2 micrograms/mL.
- Administer with caution with other ototoxic drugs such as furosemide or ethacrynic acid.
- Administer with caution with other nephrotoxic drugs such as cisplatin or cephalosporins.

- Advise the female client to immediately notify the prescriber of known or suspected pregnancy.
- Administer with caution to clients with neuromuscular disorders such as myasthenia gravis or Parkinson's disease because the drug may worsen these conditions.
- Advise client to drink plenty of fluids during therapy.
- Do not apply topical forms to large denuded body surfaces due to possible drug absorption.

Generic: glimepiride (gly-MEP-ur-ide)

Brand: Amaryl

Classification(s): Antidiabetic; hormone; sulfonylurea

Side Effects: Hypoglycemia, dizziness, asthenia, headache, nausea, increased risk of cardiovascular mortality

Nursing Implications and Precautions:

- Do not administer to clients with ketoacidosis (this should be treated with insulin).

- Assess for history of allergy to sulfonamides.

- Monitor serum glucose and assess for hypoglycemia during therapy.

- Administer with caution to clients with impaired renal or hepatic function, adrenal or pituitary insufficiency, or debilitated clients.

- Advise client of the importance of adhering to all exercise, weight control, and dietary instructions provided by the prescriber.

- Teach client to recognize signs of hypoglycemia and to keep a source of sugar available in the event symptoms occur.

- Advise client to monitor serum glucose levels more frequently during infections or periods of stress or heavy exercise.

- Advise client to take drug exactly as prescribed and not to discontinue the drug or change the dose without consulting with the prescriber.

- Advise client not to concurrently take nonsteroidal anti-inflammatory drugs unless approved by the prescriber.

Generic: glipizide (GLIP-ih-zide)

Brand: Glucotrol

Classification(s): Antidiabetic; sulfonylurea

Side Effects: Nausea, diarrhea, hypoglycemia, allergic skin reactions, dizziness, headache, increased risk of cardiovascular mortality

Nursing Implications and Precautions:

- Do not administer to clients with ketoacidosis (this should be treated with insulin).

- Assess for history of allergy to sulfonamides.

- Monitor serum glucose and assess for hypoglycemia during therapy.

- Administer with caution to clients with impaired renal or hepatic function, adrenal or pituitary insufficiency, or debilitated clients.

- Advise client of the importance of adhering to all exercise, weight control, and dietary instructions provided by the prescriber.

- Teach client to recognize signs of hypoglycemia and to keep a source of sugar available in the event symptoms occur.

- Advise client to monitor serum glucose levels more frequently during infections or periods of stress or heavy exercise.

- Advise client to take drug exactly as prescribed and not to discontinue the drug or change the dose without consulting with the prescriber.

- Advise client not to concurrently take nonsteroidal anti-inflammatory drugs unless approved by the prescriber.

- Advise clients taking extended-release forms to swallow the drug whole and not to crush, split, or chew the tablets.

Generic: glyburide (GLY-byour-ide)

Brand: DiaBeta, Micronase, Glynase

Classification(s): Antidiabetic; sulfonylurea

Side Effects: Nausea, diarrhea, hypoglycemia, allergic skin reactions, dizziness, headache, cholestatic jaundice, increased risk of cardiovascular mortality

Nursing Implications and Precautions:

- Do not administer to clients with ketoacidosis (this should be treated with insulin).

- Assess for history of allergy to sulfonamides.

- Monitor serum glucose and assess for hypoglycemia during therapy.

- Administer with caution to clients with impaired renal or hepatic function, adrenal or pituitary insufficiency, or debilitated clients.

- Advise client of the importance of adhering to all exercise, weight control, and dietary instructions provided by the prescriber.

- Teach client to recognize signs of hypoglycemia and to keep a source of sugar available in the event symptoms occur.

- Advise client to monitor serum glucose levels more frequently during infections or periods of stress or heavy exercise.

- Advise client to take drug exactly as prescribed and not to discontinue the drug or change the dose without consulting with the prescriber.

- Advise client not to concurrently take nonsteroidal anti-inflammatory drugs unless approved by the prescriber.

- Advise clients taking extended-release forms to swallow the drug whole and not to crush, split, or chew the tablets.

- Monitor hepatic function and discontinue if jaundice occurs.

Generic: heparin (HEP-uh-rin)

Brand: generic only

Classification(s): Anticoagulant

Side Effects: Hemorrhage, heparin-induced thrombocytopenia (HIT), local injection site reactions, hypersensitivity reactions, elevated aminotransferase levels

Nursing Implications and Precautions:

- Do not administer to clients with severe thrombocytopenia or uncontrollable active bleeding (except if due to disseminated intravascular coagulation).

- Do not administer by the intramuscular route.

- Administer with caution to clients who are bleeding or who have conditions with increased risk of hemorrhage (such as surgery, bacterial endocarditis, or severe hypertension).

- Monitor periodic blood coagulation tests, platelet, hematocrit, and for occult blood in stool.

- Do not administer heparin solutions containing the preservative benzyl alcohol to neonates.

- Administer with caution to clients concurrently taking anticoagulants or antiplatelet drugs.

- Carefully examine all heparin medication vials and double check all doses because fatal medication errors have occurred with this drug.

Generic: hydrochlorothiazide (HYE-droh-klor-oh-THIGH-ah-zide)

Brand: Microzide

Classification(s): Thiazide diuretic; electrolytic and water balance agent

Side Effects: Electrolyte disorders (especially hypokalemia), hyperglycemia, hyperuricemia, photosensitivity, orthostatic hypotension, GI disturbances, adverse lipid values

Nursing Implications and Precautions:

- Do not administer to clients with anuria or sulfonamide allergy.

- Administer with caution to clients with renal or hepatic dysfunction, diabetes, gout, asthma, lupus, or parathyroid disease.

- Monitor blood pressure, electrolytes, and blood urea nitrogen (BUN); discontinue if electrolyte disorders develop rapidly.

- Administer potassium supplements as prescribed.

- Monitor periodic blood glucose levels in clients with diabetes.

- Advise client to limit or eliminate alcohol use during therapy because this increases the risk of orthostatic hypotension.

- Advise client to avoid becoming overheated or dehydrated while exercising.

- Advise client to have blood pressure checked at regular intervals.

Generic: hydrocodone with acetaminophen (APAP)
(high-droh-KOH-doan)

Brand: Lorcet, others

Classification(s): Antipyretic; nonnarcotic analgesic

Side Effects: Respiratory depression, light-headedness, sedation, nausea and vomiting, dysphoria, constipation

Nursing Implications and Precautions:

- Monitor carefully in clients with high potential for substance abuse.

- Do not administer to clients with head injury or high intracranial pressure.

- Monitor for interactions with other CNS depressants.

- Monitor for excessive sedation.

- Advise client to avoid driving and other hazardous activities until the effects of the drug are known.

- Advise client to limit or eliminate alcohol use during therapy because this may cause excessive drowsiness.

- Do not administer to clients with paralytic ileus, acute or severe asthma, or severe respiratory depression.

- Administer with caution in clients with a history of drug abuse.

- With high doses of acetaminophen, monitor for hepatotoxicity.

Generic: hydrocortisone (HIGH-droh-KORT-ah-sone)

Brand: Cortef, Hydrocortone, Solu-Cortef

Classification(s): Anti-inflammatory; immunosuppressant; adrenocortical steroid

Side Effects: Adrenal insufficiency/atrophy, Cushing's syndrome, masking of active infection, glaucoma, cataracts, secondary infections, electrolyte deficiencies, hypertension, behavioral changes, osteoporosis, peptic ulcer, dermal atrophy, carbohydrate intolerance

Nursing Implications and Precautions:

- Do not administer to clients with systemic mycoses or other severe infections.
- Do not administer immunizations with live vaccines during therapy.
- Administer with caution to clients with any viral, bacterial, fungal, or protozoal infection.
- Administer with caution to clients with hypothyroidism, hepatic cirrhosis, renal insufficiency, peptic ulcer, hypertension, osteoporosis, or diabetes.
- Advise client to take drug exactly as prescribed and not to discontinue the drug or change the dose without consulting with the prescriber.

- Monitor weight, growth, and fluid and electrolyte balance.
- Do not administer topical forms to large surface areas or use occlusive dressings.
- Monitor blood pressure during prolonged therapy.
- Advise client to notify prescriber of any unusual stress, serious illness, fever, or infection because doses may need to be increased during these periods.
- Advise clients to avoid crowds or places where they may be exposed to people with infections.

Generic: hydroxychloroquine (hye-DROX-ee-KLOR-oh-kwin)

Brand: Plaquenil

Classification(s): Antimalarial; antirheumatic; biologic response modifier; disease-modifying rheumatic drug (DMARD)

Generic: hydroxyzine (high-DROX-ee-zeen)

Brand: Vistaril

Classification(s): Antihistamine; antipruritic; antianxiety; antiemetic; H_1-receptor antagonist

Side Effects: Retinopathy, blurred vision, corneal edema or deposits, visual field defects, neuromuscular dysfunction, pruritus, skin pigmentation, rash, blood dyscrasias, anorexia, nausea, weight loss

Nursing Implications and Precautions:

- Do not administer for long-term use in children to clients with retinal or visual field changes.

- Advise client to store in a safe place because this drug is very toxic to children.

- Monitor periodic blood counts and discontinue if a blood dyscrasia develops.

- Monitor for changes in vision and immediately discontinue if symptoms develop.

- Assess for ankle and knee reflexes during therapy and discontinue if muscle weakness develops.

- If treating rheumatoid arthritis or lupus, assess for symptoms and discontinue drug if no improvement is measured after 6 months of therapy.

- Administer with caution to clients with psoriasis, porphyria, hepatic dysfunction, alcoholism, or G6PD deficiency.

- Administer with caution with other hepatotoxic or dermatotoxic drugs.

Side Effects: Drowsiness, dry mouth, tremor, convulsions

Nursing Implications and Precautions:

- Administer with caution concurrently with CNS depressants because excessive drowsiness may result.

- Advise client to avoid driving and other hazardous activities until the effects of the drug are known.

- Advise client to limit or eliminate alcohol use during therapy because this may cause excessive drowsiness.

Generic: ibandronate (eye-BAN-droh-nate)

Brand: Boniva

Classification(s): Bone metabolism regulator; bisphosphonate

Side Effects: Diarrhea, nausea, headache, musculoskeletal pain, pathologic fractures, osteonecrosis of the jaw

Nursing Implications and Precautions:

- Do not administer to clients with abnormalities of the esophagus that could delay esophageal emptying.

- Do not administer to clients with hypocalcemia.

- Administer drug with plain water, preferably 1–2 hours before breakfast.

- Ensure that client remains upright for at least 60 minutes after taking drug.

- Advise client to immediately report jaw pain, swelling, loose teeth, or gum infections.

- Do not administer with medicines that contain calcium, aluminum, or magnesium.

- Assess results of periodic bone mineral density tests to ensure effectiveness of therapy.

- Advise client to include adequate amounts of vitamin D and calcium in the diet.

- Assess for hypocalcemia and correct prior to starting drug therapy.

- Administer with caution concurrently with nonsteroidal anti-inflammatory drugs because this may worsen gastrointestinal irritation.

Generic: ibuprofen (eye-byoo-PROH-fen)

Brand: Motrin, others

Classification(s): Analgesic, nonsteroidal anti-inflammatory drug (NSAID) (COX-1 and COX-2 inhibitor); antipyretic

Side Effects: Gastrointestinal (GI) ulceration or bleeding, abdominal pain, diarrhea, dyspepsia, peripheral edema, dizziness, rash, increased risk of thrombotic events, Stevens-Johnson syndrome, allergic reactions

Nursing Implications and Precautions:

- Monitor client during therapy for thrombotic events, myocardial infarction, and stroke.

- Do not administer drug for the treatment or peripoperative pain in the setting of coronary artery bypass graft surgery.

- Monitor client during therapy for GI bleeding.

- Administer with caution in clients with a history of peptic ulcers or gastrointestinal bleeding, heart failure, hypertension, or renal impairment.

- Monitor laboratory results for liver function; discontinue drug and notify prescriber if abnormal liver enzymes persist or worsen.

- Advise client to immediately report rash, blistering of the skin, or flu symptoms.

- Monitor for abnormal bleeding in clients taking warfarin because concurrent use may increase the risk of bleeding.

- Advise client to immediately report signs of hepatotoxicity (nausea, fatigue, jaundice, right upper quadrant pain).

- Monitor blood pressure regularly during therapy.

- Assess for history of hypersensitivity to nonsteroidal anti-inflammatory drugs.

- Advise clients to not administer to children for more than 2 days or to children under 3 years of age without physician approval.

Generic: insulin (IN-sule-in)

Brand: Novolin, others

Classification(s): Short-acting insulin; antidiabetic

Side Effects: Hypoglycemia, hypokalemia, overdose (hypoglycemia, coma, seizure), injection site reaction, lipodystrophy, pruritus, rash, allergy

Nursing Implications and Precautions:

- Teach client how and when to correctly self-administer insulin.
- Advise client to store insulin exactly as directed by the prescriber.
- Advise client to take drug exactly as prescribed and not to discontinue the drug or change the dose without consulting with the prescriber.
- Monitor serum glucose regularly, especially at the beginning of therapy and when dosage is adjusted.
- Teach client to recognize signs of hypoglycemia and to keep a source of sugar available in the event symptoms occur.

- Teach client to recognize signs of hyperglycemia.
- Rotate injection sites to prevent adverse skin reactions.
- Advise client to carry an identification card or wear a medical alert bracelet indicating the presence of diabetes.
- Advise client not to skip meals.
- Advise client to use disposable needles only once, and to dispose of them properly.
- Advise client to check blood sugar more frequently during periods of stress, illness, or exercise.

Generic: ipratropium (EYE-prah-TROH-pee-um)

Brand: Atrovent, Combivent

Classification(s): Bronchodilator; anticholinergic; antimuscarinic

Side Effects: Paradoxical bronchospasm, nervousness, headache, palpitations, local irritation, dry mouth, epistaxis (nasal spray form), allergy

Nursing Implications and Precautions:

- Do not administer drug with Atrovent inhaler to clients with allergy to soya lecithin or peanuts.

- If using an inhaler, teach client proper use of the device.

- Advise client that this drug should not be used to treat an acute asthma attack that has already begun.

- Administer with caution to clients with narrow-angle glaucoma or urinary retention.

- Advise client to take drug exactly as prescribed and not use larger doses without consulting with the prescriber.

- Advise client to keep track of the number of sprays used and to obtain refills before 200 sprays are reached.

- Advise client to continue taking the drug, even if feeling better.

Generic: **irbesartan** (err-bee-SAR-tan)

Brand: Avapro

Classification(s): Antihypertensive; angiotensin II receptor antagonist

Side Effects: Diarrhea, dyspepsia, fatigue, rhabdomyolysis (rare), fetal death and injury

Nursing Implications and Precautions:

- Instruct women of childbearing age to use effective birth control method (pregnancy Category D in second and third trimesters).

- Advise the female client to immediately notify the prescriber of known or suspected pregnancy.

- Monitor blood pressure during therapy to evaluate drug effectiveness.

- Advise client to take drug for the entire length of time prescribed, even if feeling better.

- Assess electrolytes and correct salt or volume depletion prior to starting therapy.

- Administer with caution to clients with renal impairment, heart failure, or renal artery stenosis.

- Advise client not to use salt substitutes containing potassium, unless directed by the prescriber.

- Monitor for myopathy and discontinue drug if symptoms of muscle pain or weakness persist.

Generic: isoniazid (eye-sow-NYE-ah-zid)

Brand: INH, Nydrazid

Classification(s): Antituberculosis; anti-infective

Side Effects: Peripheral neuropathy, hepatic injury, nausea/vomiting, blood dyscrasias, pyridoxine deficiency, hyperglycemia, rheumatic and SLE-like syndrome

Nursing Implications and Precautions:

- Do not administer to clients with severe liver disease.

- Administer with caution to clients with impaired renal or hepatic function, alcoholism, or diabetes.

- Advise client to immediately report signs of liver disease during therapy (persistent nausea/vomiting, severe stomach pain, unusual fatigue, dark urine, yellowing eyes/skin).

- Monitor hepatic enzymes regularly in older adult clients because this population has an increased risk of serious liver damage from the drug.

- Advise client to limit or eliminate alcohol use during therapy because this increases the risk for hepatitis.

- Administer with pyridoxine supplements (vitamin B_6), as necessary.

- Administer on an empty stomach because food significantly inhibits drug absorption.

- Advise client to continue taking the drug, even if feeling better.

Generic: isosorbide mononitrate (eye-sow-SORE-bide mon-oh-NYE-trate)

Brand: IMdur, Ismo, Monoket

Classification(s): Nitrate vasodilator; antianginal

Side Effects: Headache, dizziness, orthostatic hypotension, bradycardia, GI upset, syncope

Nursing Implications and Precautions:

- Do not administer concurrently with sildenafil or similar drugs because this may cause severe hypotension.

- Administer with caution to clients with acute myocardial infarction, heart failure, hypotension, volume depletion, or hypertrophic cardiomyopathy.

- Monitor for tolerance to the effects of the drug.

- Advise client to move slowly from a lying to a standing position to prevent light-headedness.

- Advise client to continue taking the drug, even if feeling better.

- Advise client to limit or eliminate alcohol use during therapy.

- Advise client that this drug should not be used to treat an acute angina attack.

- Advise client to not discontinue the drug abruptly because this may precipitate angina pain.

- Administer drug in the morning after getting out of bed.

- Advise client not to crush or chew the extended-release tablet.

Generic: lamotrigene (lam-MOW-trih-jeen)

Brand: Lamictal

Classification(s): Anticonvulsant

Side Effects: Dizziness, ataxia, fatigue, headache, vision changes, nausea/vomiting, blood dyscrasias, acute multiorgan failure, Stevens-Johnson syndrome (rare), suicidal ideation

Nursing Implications and Precautions:

- Monitor for rash and discontinue drug if rash develops.

- Avoid rapid dose increases and exceeding recommended dose because these increase the risk of serious rash.

- Administer with caution to clients with a history of allergy or rash to other antiepileptic drugs, impaired cardiac function, hepatic impairment, renal impairment, or suicidal ideation.

- Advise client to not discontinue the drug abruptly because seizures may result.

- Monitor for mood disorders, worsening depression, and suicidal ideation.

- Monitor for vision changes.

- Administer with caution to clients concurrently taking valproate because this increases the toxicity of lamotrigene.

- Administer with caution to clients concurrently taking oral contraceptives, carbamazepine, phenytoin, or rifampin because these decrease lamotrigene levels, which may precipitate seizures.

Generic: lansoprazole (lan-SOH-prah-zole)

Brand: Prevacid

Classification(s): Antiulcer; antisecretory; proton pump inhibitor

Generic: latanoprost ophthalmic (la-TAN-oh-prost off-THALL-mik)

Brand: Xalatan

Classification(s): Prostaglandin; eye preparation

Side Effects: Headache, diarrhea, abdominal pain, nausea, constipation

Nursing Implications and Precautions:

- Administer with caution with drugs for which gastric pH affects bioavailability (such as ketoconazole, iron salts, and digoxin).
- Administer drug at least 1 hour before a meal.
- Advise clients taking extended-release forms to swallow the drug whole and not to crush, split, or chew the capsules.
- Advise client to continue taking the drug for the entire length of time prescribed, even if feeling better.
- Advise client to notify the prescriber if symptoms have not resolved following 4–8 weeks of therapy.
- Do not administer concurrently with atazanavir.
- Administer with caution to clients with severe hepatic impairment.

Side Effects: Increased ocular pigmentation, blurred vision, burning, stinging, local conjunctival hyperemia, sensation of foreign body in the eye, itching, punctate epithelial keratopathy

Nursing Implications and Precautions:

- Advise client to not exceed the prescribed dose because this may reduce the drug's effectiveness.
- Administer with caution to clients with ocular inflammation, aphakia, pseudophakia with torn posterior lens capsule, or those with a risk for macular edema.
- Advise client to remove contact lenses before using the drug and to wait at least 15 minutes before reinsertion.
- Advise client to wait at least 5 minutes between applications of other topical ophthalmic drugs.
- Advise client that the drug may change the color of the eyes, eyelashes, or eyelids, as well as increased growth of the eyelashes.
- Teach client proper method of instilling drug on the eye.

Generic: levodopa (lev-oh-DOPE-uh)

Brand: Larodopa

Classification(s): Antiparkinson; dopamine receptor agonist

Side Effects: Dyskinesias, nausea/vomiting, behavioral changes, arrythmias, hypotension, headache, dizziness

Nursing Implications and Precautions:

- Do not administer this drug to clients with narrow-angle glaucoma, undiagnosed skin lesions, melanoma, or those taking monoamine oxidase (MAO) inhibitors.

- Administer with caution to clients with severe cardiovascular or pulmonary disease, asthma, renal, hepatic, or endocrine disorders, history of peptic ulcer or myocardial infarction with residual arrhythmias, suicidal ideation, psychosis, orthostatic hypotension, or chronic wide-angle glaucoma.

- Discontinue levodopa at least 12 hours before starting Sinemet.

- Monitor renal and hepatic function, intraocular pressure, and blood counts during therapy.

- Monitor for dyskinesias, which may require dose reduction.

- Monitor for mood disorders, psychosis, and suicidal ideation.

- Advise client to report any new skin lesions during therapy because this drug increases the risk for melanoma.

- Use caution when administering concurrently with phenothiazines or risperidone because these reduce the effectiveness of levodopa.

Generic: levofloxacin (leev-oh-FLOX-ah-sin)

Brand: Levaquin

Classification(s): Antibiotic, quinolone

Generic: levothyroxine (lee-voh-thy-ROX-in)

Brand: Levothroid, others

Classification(s): Thyroid hormone replacement

Side Effects: Nausea, vomiting, headache, dizziness, insomnia, constipation, tendinitis, tendon rupture, allergic reactions, photosensitivity, hepatotoxicity

Nursing Implications and Precautions:

- Advise client to take drug for the entire length of time prescribed, even if symptoms of infection have resolved.

- Assess for history of hypersensitivity to fluoroquinolones or other antibiotics.

- Monitor for tendonitis or tendon rupture.

- Advise client to immediately report any unusual pain, or inflammation or swelling of joints, especially the Achilles tendon.

- Monitor for pseudomembranous colitis (severe diarrhea).

- Advise client to minimize exposure to direct sunlight and to wear protective clothing if exposed to the sun.

- Do not administer sucralfate or antacids containing magnesium or aluminum within 2 hours of a dose of levofloxacin.

- Advise client to not take drug with dairy products or with calcium-fortified juice.

- Monitor liver enzyme tests for possible hepatotoxicity.

Side Effects: Hyperthyroidism (nervousness, tachycardia, insomnia, anxiety, sweating, weight loss), menstrual irregularities

Nursing Implications and Precautions:

- Monitor carefully for signs of hyperthyroidism.

- Assess for decreased bone mineral density.

- Should not be administered for the treatment of obesity or weight loss.

- Administer with caution to clients with cardiovascular disease.

- Monitor laboratory tests for thyroid function.

Generic: lidocaine topical (LYE-doe-caine)

Brand: Lidoderm

Classification(s): Antiarrhythmic, class IB; local anesthetic; anticonvulsant

Generic: lisinopril (lye-SIN-oh-prill)

Brand: Prinivil, Zestril

Classification(s): Antihypertensive; angiotensin-converting enzyme (ACE) inhibitor

Side Effects: Local erythema and edema, allergic reactions (urticaria, angioedema, bronchospasm)

Nursing Implications and Precautions:

- Do not apply to large areas of denuded or inflamed skin.
- When applying the drug, avoid eyes or mucous membranes.
- Administer with caution if using long duration of application or more than three patches in 24 hours.
- Advise client that the drug (and the used patch) is toxic to children and pets.
- Administer with caution to clients with hepatic disease.
- Remove patch if irritation or burning occurs; do not reapply until irritation subsides.
- Do not apply to clients who are allergic to amide-type local anesthetics.

Side Effects: Headache, cough, dizziness, orthostatic hypotension, angioedema, fetal death and injury

Nursing Implications and Precautions:

- Instruct women of childbearing age to use effective birth control method (pregnancy Category D).
- Advise the female client to immediately notify the prescriber of known or suspected pregnancy.
- Use with caution in clients with kidney or liver disease.
- Advise client to limit or eliminate alcohol use during therapy.
- Monitor blood pressure during therapy to evaluate drug effectiveness.
- Advise client to move slowly from a lying to a standing position to prevent light-headedness.
- Advise client to drink at least 6–8 glasses of water each day.
- Advise client to take drug for the entire length of time prescribed.
- Advise client not to use salt substitutes containing potassium, unless directed by the prescriber.

Generic: lithium (LITH-ee-um)

Brand: Eskalith, Lithobid

Classification(s): Antipsychotic; antimanic; antidepressant; mood stabilizer

Side Effects: Polyuria, polydipsia, drowsiness, tremor, hypothyroidism, extrapyramidal symptoms, GI upset, renal toxicity, seizures, arrhythmias, hypotension, lethargy, metallic taste, dry mouth, blurred vision, pseudotumor cerebri, fetal injury

Nursing Implications and Precautions:

- Do not administer to clients with renal or cardiovascular disease, sodium depletion, or who are severely debilitated or dehydrated.

- Monitor clients closely who are concurrently taking diuretics.

- Administer with caution to clients with seizure disorders.

- Monitor fluid and salt intake, especially in clients with fever, sweating, diarrhea, or infection.

- Monitor serum lithium levels frequently because the toxic and therapeutic levels are very close.

- Monitor thyroid and renal function during therapy.

- Discontinue drug if diarrhea, vomiting, tremor, ataxia, drowsiness, or weakness occur.

- Instruct women of childbearing age to use effective birth control method (pregnancy Category D).

- Advise client to notify health care providers of all medications taken because lithium interacts with multiple drugs.

- Advise client to immediately notify the prescriber if clinical signs of lithium toxicity occur: diarrhea, vomiting, tremor, mild ataxia, drowsiness, or muscular weakness.

Generic: lorazepam (lor-AZE-ah-pam)

Brand: Ativan

Classification(s): Antianxiety; sedative-hypnotic; benzodiazepine

Side Effects: Dizziness, ataxia, drowsiness, sedation, confusion, dependence, blurred vision, seizures, birth defects (pregnancy Category D)

Nursing Implications and Precautions:

- Advise client to not discontinue the drug abruptly.
- Advise client to avoid driving and other hazardous activities until the effects of the drug are known.
- Do not administer to clients with suicidal ideation.
- Assess for signs of overdose or abuse (confusion, sedation, slurred speech, coma).
- Advise client to store drug in a safe place, away from children or those who may take the drug for recreational purposes.
- Advise the female client to immediately notify the prescriber of known or suspected pregnancy.
- Advise client to limit or eliminate alcohol use during therapy.
- Use caution when administering other CNS depressants concurrently with lorazepam due to the potential for excessive sedation.

Generic: losartan (low-SAR-tan)

Brand: Hyzaar

Classification(s): Antihypertensive; angiotensin II receptor antagonist

Side Effects: Diarrhea, abdominal pain. dyspepsia, fatigue, rhabdomyolysis (rare), fetal death and injury, upper respiratory tract infection

Nursing Implications and Precautions:

- Instruct women of childbearing age to use effective birth control method (pregnancy Category D in second and third trimesters).

- Advise the female client to immediately notify the prescriber of known or suspected pregnancy.

- Monitor blood pressure during therapy to evaluate drug effectiveness.

- Advise client to take drug for the entire length of time prescribed, even if feeling better.

- Assess electrolytes and correct salt or volume depletion prior to starting therapy.

- Administer with caution to clients with hypovolemia, renal or hepatic impairment, diabetes, asthma, heart failure, or renal artery stenosis.

- Advise client not to use salt substitutes containing potassium, unless directed by the prescriber.

- Monitor for myopathy and discontinue drug if symptoms of muscle pain or weakness persist.

Generic: lovastatin (low-vah-STAT-in)

Brand: Altoprev, Mevacor

Classification(s): Antilipemic; statin; HMG-CoA reductase inhibitor

Generic: meclizine (MEK-lih-zeen)

Brand: Antivert

Classification(s): Antihistamine; antivertigo; H_1-receptor antagonist

Side Effects: Intestinal cramping, diarrhea, constipation, nasopharyngitis, arthralgia, myopathy

Nursing Implications and Precautions:

- Monitor liver enzymes during therapy for possible hepatotoxicity.
- Do not administer to clients with active liver disease.
- Assess for myopathy (muscle pain and weakness).
- Administer with caution concurrently with strong CYP3A4 enzyme inhibitors (such as clarithromycin, azole antifungals, grapefruit juice, or cyclosporine).
- Instruct women of childbearing age to use effective birth control method (pregnancy Category X).
- Advise client to continue taking the drug, even if feeling better.
- Administer drug at least 1 hour before or at least 4 hours after taking bile acid-binding resins such as cholestyramine or colestipol.
- Advise clients taking extended-release forms to swallow the drug whole and not to crush, split, or chew the capsules.
- Advise client to limit or eliminate alcohol use during therapy because this increases the risk for hepatic toxicity.

Side Effects: Drowsiness, anticholinergic effects (dry mouth, dizziness, blurred vision, nausea)

Nursing Implications and Precautions:

- Administer with caution to clients with asthma, glaucoma, prostate enlargement, or gastrointestinal obstruction.
- Advise client to avoid driving and other hazardous activities until the effects of the drug are known.
- Advise client to limit or eliminate alcohol use during therapy because this may cause excessive drowsiness.
- If taken for motion sickness, administer 1 hour before expected travel.

Generic: meloxicam (mell-OX-ee-cam)

Brand: Mobic

Classification(s): Antirheumatic; antipyretic; analgesic, nonsteroidal anti-inflammatory drug (NSAID)

Generic: memantine (meh-MAN-teen)

Brand: Namenda

Classification(s): Antidementia; anti-Alzheimer's; *N*-methyl-D-aspartate (NMDA) receptor antagonist

Side Effects: Gastrointestinal (GI) ulceration or bleeding, abdominal pain, diarrhea, dyspepsia, peripheral edema, dizziness, rash, increased risk of thrombotic events, Stevens-Johnson syndrome, allergic reactions

Nursing Implications and Precautions:

- Monitor client during therapy for thrombotic events, myocardial infarction, and stroke.
- Do not administer drug for the treatment of peripoperative pain in the setting of coronary artery bypass graft surgery.
- Monitor client during therapy for GI bleeding.
- Administer with caution in clients with a history of peptic ulcers or gastrointestinal bleeding, heart failure, hypertension, or renal impairment.
- Monitor laboratory results for liver function; discontinue drug and notify prescriber if abnormal liver enzymes persist or worsen.
- Advise client to immediately report rash, blistering of the skin, or flu symptoms.
- Monitor for abnormal bleeding in clients taking warfarin because concurrent use may increase the risk of bleeding.
- Advise client to immediately report signs of hepatotoxicity (nausea, fatigue, jaundice, right upper quadrant pain).
- Monitor blood pressure regularly during therapy.
- Assess for history of hypersensitivity to nonsteroidal anti-inflammatory drugs.

Side Effects: Headache, dizziness, GI upset, constipation, hypertension, back pain, somnolence, hallucination

Nursing Implications and Precautions:

- Administer with caution to clients with severe hepatic impairment, alkalinized urine, and seizure disorders.
- Advise client to avoid driving and other hazardous activities until the effects of the drug are known.
- Advise client to continue taking the drug, even if feeling better.

Generic: **metaxalone** (me-TAX-ah-lone)

Brand: Skelaxin

Classification(s): Muscle relaxant

Side Effects: Drowsiness, dizziness, headache, nervousness, nausea/vomiting, rash, jaundice, hemolytic anemia, leukopenia, hypersensitivity reactions

Nursing Implications and Precautions:

- Do not administer to clients with anemias or significant renal or hepatic impairment.

- Administer with caution to clients with hepatic dysfunction and monitor liver enzymes during therapy.

- Advise client that use with alcohol or other CNS depressants may cause excessive drowsiness.

- Advise client to avoid driving and other hazardous activities until the effects of the drug are known.

- Administer with caution in older adult clients because they experience a higher incidence of CNS side effects.

Generic: metformin (met-FOR-min)

Brand: Glucophage

Classification(s): Antihyperglycemic; antidiabetic; biguanide

Side Effects: GI disturbances, taste disturbance, lactic acidosis (rare)

Nursing Implications and Precautions:

- Do not administer to clients with significant renal impairment, metabolic acidosis, or ketoacidosis.

- Discontinue drug during the administration of intravascular iodinated contrast agents and for 48 hours afterwards.

- Assess for normal renal function before initiating therapy and monitor renal status during therapy.

- Administer with caution to clients with hepatic impairment, deficient caloric intake, adrenal or pituitary insufficiency, or alcohol intoxication.

- Discontinue drug if lactic acidosis, shock, acute MI, sepsis, or hypoxemia occurs.

- Assess for dehydration and discontinue drug if this occurs.

- Monitor hepatic function and hematology.

- Advise client to monitor serum glucose levels more frequently during infections or periods of stress or heavy exercise.

- Teach client to recognize signs of hypoglycemia and to keep a source of sugar available in the event symptoms occur.

- Advise clients taking extended-release forms to swallow the drug whole and not to crush, split, or chew the tablets.

- Administer with vitamin B_{12} supplements, as necessary.

- Monitor for symptoms of lactic acidosis (weakness, increasing sleepiness, slow heart rate, cold feeling, muscle pain, shortness of breath, stomach pain, feeling light-headed, and fainting.)

Generic: methadone (METH-ah-doan)

Brand: Dolophine, others

Classification(s): Narcotic (opiate agonist) analgesic; toxicology agent

Generic: methocarbamol (METH-oh-KARB-ah-mall)

Brand: Robaxin

Classification(s): Central-acting skeletal muscle relaxant; carbamate

Side Effects: Respiratory depression, light-headedness, sedation, nausea and vomiting, dysphoria, constipation

Nursing Implications and Precautions:

- Advise client to store drug in a safe place, away from children or those who may take the drug for recreational purposes.

- When used to treat narcotic dependence, monitor compliance carefully to determine if the client is taking the drug in the prescribed manner.

- Do not administer to clients with head injury or high intracranial pressure.

- Monitor for interactions with other CNS depressants.

- Monitor for excessive sedation.

- Advise client to avoid driving and other hazardous activities until the effects of the drug are known.

- Advise client to limit or eliminate alcohol use during therapy because this may cause excessive drowsiness.

- Do not administer to clients with paralytic ileus, acute or severe asthma, or severe respiratory depression.

- Monitor the electrocardiogram for evidence of QT interval prolongation.

Side Effects: Drowsiness, dizziness, nausea/vomiting, blurred vision, headache

Nursing Implications and Precautions:

- Do not administer to clients with pre-existing acidosis and urea retention with renal impairment.

- Advise client to avoid driving and other hazardous activities until the effects of the drug are known.

- Advise client that use with alcohol or other CNS depressants may cause excessive drowsiness.

- Advise client to take drug exactly as prescribed and not to take it more frequently.

Generic: methotrexate (meth-oh-TREX-ate)

Brand: Rheumatrex

Classification(s): Antineoplastic; antifolate; antirheumatic; antipsoriatic; antimetabolite; immunosuppressant; disease-modifying antirheumatic drug (DMARD)

Side Effects: Hepatotoxicity, nausea/vomiting, stomatitis, blood dyscrasias, rash, pruritus, dermatitis, diarrhea, alopecia, dizziness, hepatoxicity, bone marrow suppression, GI toxicity, tumor lysis syndrome, fatal skin reactions, opportunistic infections, pulmonary toxicity, fetal toxicity (pregnancy Category X)

Nursing Implications and Precautions:

- Do not administer to clients with immunodeficiency, blood dyscrasias, alcoholism, chronic liver disease, or during pregnancy.

- Monitor for malignant lymphomas and discontinue drug if they occur.

- Prior to starting therapy, obtain complete blood count (CBCs) with differential, chest X-ray, and assess hepatic, renal, and pulmonary function.

- Monitor hematology, renal, and hepatic function regularly during therapy. Discontinue immediately if blood counts drop significantly.

- Prior to starting therapy, rule out pregnancy in women of childbearing potential and advise these clients to use effective contraception during therapy.

- Monitor for vomiting, diarrhea, stomatitis, or pulmonary symptoms and interrupt therapy if these occur.

- Administer with caution in clients with hepatic and renal impairment, obesity, diabetes, peptic ulcer, ulcerative colitis active, infection, dehydration, folate deficiency, ascites, and pleural effusions.

- Administer with caution concurrently with hepatotoxic or nephrotoxic drugs.

- Advise client to notify health care providers of all medications taken because methotrexate interacts with multiple drugs.

Generic: methylphenidate (meth-il-FEN-uh-date)

Brand: Concerta, Ritalin, Metadate, Methylin

Classification(s): Cerebral stimulant

Side Effects: Decreased appetite, headache, dry mouth, nausea, insomnia, anxiety, dizziness, weight loss, irritability, hyperhidrosis, hypertension, visual disturbances

Nursing Implications and Precautions:

- Do not administer this drug within 2 weeks of taking monoamine oxidase (MAO) inhibitors.

- Do not administer this drug to clients with serious anxiety, agitation, glaucoma, motor tics, or Tourette's syndrome.

- Administer with caution in clients with heart disease, recent myocardial infarction, hypertension, hyperthyroidism, diabetes, psychosis, depression, seizure disorders, glaucoma, and bipolar disorder.

- Monitor for signs of excessive CNS stimulation (irritability, insomnia, nervousness, palpitations, tremor).

- In children, monitor growth and weight during therapy because this drug can suppress long-term growth.

- Advise client to store drug in a safe place, away from children or those who may take the drug for recreational purposes.

- Advise clients taking extended-release forms to swallow the drug whole and not to crush, split, or chew the capsules.

- Administer with caution in clients with a history of drug abuse.

- Administer drug early in the day, to prevent insomnia.

Generic: methylprednisolone (METH-ill-pred-NISS-oh-lone)

Brand: Medrol

Classification(s): Anti-inflammatory; biological response modifier; immunosuppressant; adrenal corticosteroid

Side Effects: Adrenal insufficiency/atrophy, Cushing's syndrome, masking of active infection, glaucoma, cataracts, secondary infections, electrolyte deficiencies, hypertension, behavioral changes, osteoporosis, peptic ulcer, dermal atrophy, carbohydrate intolerance

Nursing Implications and Precautions:

- Do not administer to clients with systemic mycoses or other severe infections.

- Do not administer immunizations with live vaccines during therapy.

- Administer with caution to clients with any viral, bacterial, fungal, or protozoal infection.

- Administer with caution to clients with hypothyroidism. hepatic cirrhosis, renal insufficiency, peptic ulcer, hypertension, osteoporosis, or diabetes.

- Advise client to take drug exactly as prescribed and not to discontinue the drug or change the dose without consulting with the prescriber.

- Monitor weight, growth, and fluid and electrolyte balance.

- Do not administer topical forms to large surface areas or use occlusive dressings.

- Monitor blood pressure during prolonged therapy.

- Advise client to notify prescriber of any unusual stress, serious illness, fever, or infection because doses may need to be increased during these periods.

- Advise clients to avoid crowds or places where they may be exposed to people with infections.

Generic: metoclopramide (MET-oh-KLOE-prah-mide)

Brand: Reglan

Classification(s): GI stimulant; antiemetic

Side Effects: Restlessness, drowsiness, fatigue, extrapyramidal effects, parkinsonism, tardive dyskinesia, neuroleptic malignant syndrome, dizziness, endocrine disturbances, hypo- or hypertension, fluid retention, GI or GU disturbances, hepatotoxicity (rare)

Nursing Implications and Precautions:

- Do not administer to clients with gastrointestinal obstruction, perforation, hemorrhage, pheochromocytoma, or epilepsy.

- Do not administer concomitant with drugs that may cause extrapyramidal reactions such as phenothiazines or haloperidol.

- Do not administer this drug within 2 weeks of taking monoamine oxidase (MAO) inhibitors.

- Administer with caution to clients with Parkinson's disease, tardive dyskinesia, cirrhosis, heart failure, hypertension, or those with a history of breast cancer or depression. Advise client to avoid driving and other hazardous activities until the effects of the drug are known.

- Advise client that use with alcohol or other CNS depressants may cause excessive drowsiness.

- Advise client to immediately report any involuntary, unusual spasms, or muscle movements of the head, mouth, tongue, or neck.

Generic: metoprolol (met-OH-proh-lole)

Brand: Lopressor, Toprol XL

Classification(s): Antihypertensive; antianginal; cardioselective beta-adrenergic antagonist

Side Effects: Bradycardia, hypotension, fatigue, dizziness, diarrhea, rash, depression, hyperglycemia

Nursing Implications and Precautions:

- Do not administer to clients with severe bradycardia, heart block greater than first degree, cardiogenic shock, or decompensated heart failure.

- Monitor for worsening heart failure.

- Advise client to not discontinue the drug abruptly because this may precipitate angina pain or myocardial infarction.

- Monitor blood glucose levels in clients with diabetes.

- Administer with caution to clients with diabetes, severe hepatic impairment, hyperthyroidism, or asthma.

- Advise client to move slowly from a lying to a standing position to prevent light-headedness.

- Advise client to limit or eliminate alcohol use because this may cause excessive drowsiness.

- Advise client not to crush or chew the extended-release tablets.

Generic: metronidazole (met-row-NIDE-ah-zole)

Brand: Flagyl, MetroGel, MetroCream

Classification(s): Amebicide; antitrichomonal; antibiotic

Side Effects: Nausea, anorexia, headache, metallic taste, dysuria, cystitis, incontinence, *Candida* infections, seizures, peripheral neuropathy, neutropenia, pancreatitis (rare), local irritation (topical creams)

Nursing Implications and Precautions:

- Do not administer to pregnant women with trichomonas during the first trimester or to clients who have taken disulfiram within the previous 2 weeks.

- Administer with caution to clients with encephalopathy, seizures, severe hepatic impairment, or blood dyscrasias.

- Monitor leukocyte counts during therapy.

- Monitor for neurological symptoms and discontinue drug if they occur.

- Advise client to eliminate alcohol use during therapy and for at least 3 days after therapy has concluded.

- Advise client to take drug for the entire length of time prescribed, even if symptoms of infection have resolved.

- Administer the extended-release forms of drug on an empty stomach, at least 1 hour before or 2 hours following a meal.

Generic: minocycline (MYE-noh-SYE-kleen)

Brand: Minocin

Classification(s): Antibiotic, tetracycline

Side Effects: Photosensitivity, hepatotoxicity, GI upset (anorexia, nausea, vomiting), blood dyscrasias, fetal toxicity (pregnancy Category D), allergic reaction, teeth discoloration in children

Nursing Implications and Precautions:

- Advise client to take drug for the entire length of time prescribed, even if symptoms of infection have resolved.

- Do not administer this drug to children under age 8 because permanent teeth discoloration may occur.

- Monitor for pseudomembranous colitis (severe diarrhea).

- Advise client to minimize exposure to direct sunlight and to wear protective clothing if exposed to the sun.

- Advise the female client to immediately notify the prescriber of known or suspected pregnancy.

- Monitor blood laboratory values during therapy.

- Do not administer zinc, iron, calcium, magnesium, or aluminum within 2 hours of a dose of doxycycline.

- Advise female clients taking oral contraceptives to use an additional method of birth control because doxycycline renders these drugs less effective.

- Advise client to avoid driving and other hazardous activities until the effects of the drug are known.

- Monitor liver enzyme tests during therapy for possible hepatotoxicity.

Generic: mirtazapine (mir-TAH-zuh-peen)

Brand: Remeron

Classification(s): Tetracyclic antidepressant; antianxiety

Side Effects: Somnolence, increased appetite, weight gain, dizziness, nausea, dry mouth

Nursing Implications and Precautions:

- Do not administer this drug within 2 weeks of taking monoamine oxidase (MAO) inhibitors.

- Advise client that use with alcohol or other CNS depressants may cause excessive drowsiness.

- Administer with caution to clients with hepatic or renal impairment, diseases that affect metabolism or hemodynamic response, history of mania/hypomania, seizure disorders, suicidal ideation, history of myocardial infarction or angina, ischemic stroke, or hypovolemia.

- Monitor for unusual changes in behavior, worsening depression, and suicidal ideation.

- Advise client to not discontinue the drug abruptly.

- Advise client that the drug must be taken several weeks before the full effects of the drug are noticed.

- Advise client to limit or eliminate alcohol use during therapy because this may cause excessive drowsiness.

Generic: mometasone (moe-MET-ah-sone)

Brand: Nasonex

Classification(s): Corticosteroid

Generic: montelukast (MON-tee-LOO-kast)

Brand: Singulair

Classification(s): Bronchodilator; leukotriene receptor antagonist

Side Effects: Headache, pharyngitis, epistaxis, nasal burning, asthma symptoms, GI upset, cough

Nursing Implications and Precautions:

- Advise client to take drug for the entire length of time prescribed, even if symptoms have resolved.

- Monitor for adrenal insufficiency if client is concurrently receiving other systemic or topical corticosteroids.

- Advise client to take drug exactly as prescribed and not to take it more frequently.

- Monitor for localized *Candida* infection and other nasal mucosal changes.

- Administer with caution to clients with tuberculosis or other infections such as chickenpox, measles, or ocular herpes simplex.

- If exposed to measles or chickenpox, consider anti-infective prophylactic therapy. Monitor for growth reduction in children.

Side Effects: Upper respiratory infection, fever, headache, otitis media, pharyngitis, neuropsychiatric events

Nursing Implications and Precautions:

- Do not abruptly withdraw oral corticosteroids when switching to montelukast.

- Advise client to take the granules by mouth within 15 minutes of opening packet.

- Advise client that this drug should not be used to treat an acute asthma attack that has already begun.

- Monitor for neuropsychiatric events such as agitation, anxiety, depression, disorientation, hallucinations, insomnia, and suicidal behavior.

- Advise client that the drug must be taken several weeks before the full effects of the drug are noticed.

Generic: morphine (MOR-feen)

Brand: Astramorph

Classification(s): Narcotic (opiate agonist) analgesic

Side Effects: Respiratory depression, light-headedness, sedation, nausea and vomiting, dysphoria, constipation

Nursing Implications and Precautions:

- Monitor carefully in clients with a potential for substance abuse.

- Do not administer to clients with head injury or high intracranial pressure.

- Monitor for interactions with other CNS depressants.

- Monitor for excessive sedation.

- Advise client to avoid driving and other hazardous activities until the effects of the drug are known.

- Advise client to limit or eliminate alcohol use during therapy because this may cause excessive drowsiness.

- Do not administer to clients with paralytic ileus, acute or severe asthma, or severe respiratory depression.

- Do not administer extended-release forms to clients unless they are opioid tolerant.

Generic: moxifloxacin (MOX-ee-FLOX-ah-sin)

Brand: Avelox, others

Classification(s): Antibiotic, quinolone

Generic: mupirocin (myoo-PEER-oh-sin)

Brand: Bactroban

Classification(s): Antibiotic

Side Effects: Nausea, vomiting, dizziness, tendinitis, tendon rupture, allergic reactions, photosensitivity, ECG changes

Nursing Implications and Precautions:

- Advise client to take drug for the entire length of time prescribed, even if symptoms of infection have resolved.

- Assess for history of hypersensitivity to fluoroquinolones or other antibiotics.

- Monitor for tendonitis or tendon rupture.

- Advise client to immediately report any unusual pain, or inflammation or swelling of joints, especially the Achilles tendon.

- Monitor for pseudomembranous colitis (severe diarrhea).

- Advise client to minimize exposure to direct sunlight and to wear protective clothing if exposed to the sun.

- Do not administer sucralfate or antacids containing magnesium or aluminum within 2 hours of a dose of moxifloxacin.

- Advise client to not take drug with dairy products or with calcium-fortified juice.

- Obtain a baseline ECG and monitor for changes during therapy.

- Use caution when administering drug to clients with ongoing arrythmias or myocardial ischemia.

Side Effects: Burning, stinging, pain, itching; for nasal form, also rhinitis, pharyngitis, changes in taste

Nursing Implications and Precautions:

- Administer cream or ointment up to three times daily.

- Advise client to notify the prescriber if the symptoms of infection do not improve in 3–5 days.

- Advise client to avoid contact of the drug with the eyes.

- Dressings may be used after the drug is applied.

- Advise client to take drug for the entire length of time prescribed, even if symptoms of infection have resolved.

Generic: nabumetone (nah-BYOO-meh-tone)

Brand: Relafen

Classification(s): Analgesic, nonsteroidal anti-inflammatory drug (NSAID); antirheumatic; antipyretic

Side Effects: Gastrointestinal (GI) ulceration or bleeding, abdominal pain, diarrhea, dyspepsia, peripheral edema, dizziness, rash, increased risk of thrombotic events, Stevens-Johnson syndrome, allergic reactions

Nursing Implications and Precautions:

- Monitor client during therapy for thrombotic events, myocardial infarction, and stroke.
- Do not administer drug for the treatment or peripoperative pain in the setting of coronary artery bypass graft surgery.
- Monitor client during therapy for GI bleeding.
- Administer with caution in clients with a history of peptic ulcers or gastrointestinal bleeding, heart failure, hypertension, or renal impairment.
- Monitor laboratory results for liver function; discontinue drug and notify prescriber if abnormal liver enzymes persist or worsen.
- Advise client to immediately report rash, blistering of the skin, or flu symptoms.
- Monitor for abnormal bleeding in clients taking warfarin because concurrent use may increase the risk of bleeding.
- Advise client to immediately report signs of hepatotoxicity (nausea, fatigue, jaundice, right upper quadrant pain).
- Monitor blood pressure regularly during therapy.
- Assess for history of hypersensitivity to nonsteroidal anti-inflammatory drugs.

Generic: naproxen (nah-PROX-en)

Brand: Aleve, others

Classification(s): Analgesic, nonsteroidal anti-inflammatory drug (NSAID); antipyretic

Side Effects: Gastrointestinal (GI) ulceration or bleeding, abdominal pain, diarrhea, dyspepsia, peripheral edema, dizziness, rash, increased risk of thrombotic events, Stevens-Johnson syndrome, allergic reactions

Nursing Implications and Precautions:

- Monitor client during therapy for thrombotic events, myocardial infarction, and stroke.

- Do not administer drug for the treatment of perioperative pain in the setting of coronary artery bypass graft surgery.

- Monitor client during therapy for GI bleeding.

- Administer with caution in clients with a history of peptic ulcers or gastrointestinal bleeding, heart failure, hypertension, or renal impairment.

- Monitor laboratory results for liver function; discontinue drug and notify prescriber if abnormal liver enzymes persist or worsen.

- Advise client to immediately report rash, blistering of the skin, or flu symptoms.

- Monitor for abnormal bleeding in clients taking warfarin because concurrent use may increase the risk of bleeding.

- Advise client to immediately report signs of hepatotoxicity (nausea, fatigue, jaundice, right upper quadrant pain).

- Monitor blood pressure regularly during therapy.

- Assess for history of hypersensitivity to nonsteroidal anti-inflammatory drugs.

Generic: niacin (NYE-ah-sin)

Brand: Niaspan

Classification(s): Antilipemic; vitamin B_3

Side Effects: Flushing, dizziness, nausea/vomiting, diarrhea, pruritus, cough, abnormal liver function tests, palpitations, shortness of breath, sweating

Nursing Implications and Precautions:

- Do not administer to clients with significant hepatic impairment, unexplained elevations of serum transaminases, active peptic ulcers, or arterial bleeding.

- Administer with caution to clients with renal impairment, unstable angina, acute MI, gout, recent surgery, history of hepatobiliary disease, or peptic ulcer.

- Advise client to eliminate alcohol use during therapy because this increases the side effects of the drug.

- Do not substitute equivalent doses of immediate-release or sustained-release niacin because hepatotoxicity may occur.

- Obtain baseline serum transaminase levels and monitor regularly; discontinue drug if levels greater than three times the upper limit of normal persist or if signs of liver disease occur.

- Monitor blood glucose regularly in diabetic clients because this drug can increase blood sugar levels.

- If client is concurrently taking statins, monitor for myopathy.

- Advise client concurrently taking colestipol or cholestyramine to take them at least 4–6 hours before or after the niacin.

- Advise client taking extended-release forms to swallow the drug whole and not to crush, split, or chew the tablets or capsules.

Generic: nifedipine (nih-FED-ih-peen)

Brand: Adalat, others

Classification(s): Antihypertensive; antianginal; calcium channel blocker

Side Effects: Flushing, hypotension, headache, dizziness, peripheral edema, hepatotoxicity, heart failure, reflex tachycardia

Nursing Implications and Precautions:

- Assess for swelling of hands, feet, and ankles.
- Use with caution in clients with heart failure or hepatic impairment.
- Monitor blood pressure periodically to ensure drug effectiveness.
- Advise client to continue taking the drug, even if symptoms resolve.
- Advise clients taking extended-release forms to swallow the drug whole and not to crush, split, or chew the capsules.
- Advise client to limit or eliminate alcohol use during therapy.
- Advise client to move slowly from a lying to a standing position to prevent light-headedness.
- Monitor client carefully when beginning therapy or changing doses because this may worsen angina pain or cause a myocardial infarction.

Generic: nitrofurantoin (NYE-trow-fyour-AN-tow-in)

Brand: Furadantin, Macrodantin, Macrobid

Classification(s): Antibiotic; urinary tract anti-infective

Side Effects: Nausea/vomiting, anorexia, headache, pulmonary disorders, hepatic damage, peripheral neuropathy, hemolytic anemia, alopecia, Stevens-Johnson syndrome (rare), anaphylaxis, blood dyscrasias

Nursing Implications and Precautions:

- Do not administer to clients with anuria, oliguria, or creatinine clearance less than 60 mL/min.

- Do not administer to neonates less than 1 month of age and women who are in labor, pregnant (at term), or breastfeeding because the drug can cause hemolytic anemia in immature erythrocyte systems.

- Administer with caution to clients with renal impairment, G6PD or vitamin B deficiency, anemia, diabetes, electrolyte imbalance, or asthma.

- Monitor for pulmonary symptoms, hepatic disorders, hemolysis, or peripheral neuropathy and immediately discontinue drug if these occur.

- Monitor renal function in clients taking the drug for prolonged periods.

- Advise client to take drug for the entire length of time prescribed, even if symptoms of infection have resolved.

- Advise client to immediately report shortness of breath, chest pain, fever/chills, unusual weakness, numbness or tingling, or severe diarrhea because these may be symptoms of serious side effects.

- Advise client not to use antacids, unless directed by the prescriber.

Generic: nitroglycerin sublingual (nye-trow-GLISS-er-in)

Brand: Nitrostat, NitroQuick, Nitrolingual

Classification(s): Antianginal; nitrate vasodilator

Generic: norepinephrine (nor-ep-ih-NEF-rin)

Brand: Levophed

Classification(s): Vasopressor; cardiac inotropic; adrenergic agonist; vasoconstrictor

Side Effects: Headache, vertigo, weakness, palpitation, orthostatic hypotension, syncope, flushing, rash

Nursing Implications and Precautions:

- Do not administer to clients with early myocardial infarction, severe anemia, or increased intracranial pressure.

- Do not administer concurrently with sildenafil or similar drugs because this may cause severe hypotension.

- Administer with caution to clients with heart failure, hypotension, volume depletion, or hypertrophic cardiomyopathy.

- Advise client to not discontinue the drug abruptly because this may precipitate angina pain.

- Discontinue drug if blurred vision or dry mouth occur.

- Advise client to move slowly from a lying to a standing position to prevent light-headedness.

- Advise client to take the drug at the first sign of anginal pain and to seek emergency assistance if the pain worsens or lasts longer than 5 minutes.

- Advise the client to allow the sublingual tablet to dissolve under the tongue without chewing or swallowing whole.

- Advise client to limit or eliminate alcohol use during therapy because this will increase the side effects of the drug.

Side Effects: Restlessness, anxiety, palpitations, headache, sweating, hypertension, cerebral hemorrhage, reflex bradycardia

Nursing Implications and Precautions:

- Do not administer to clients with hypotension due to volume deficit or peripheral vascular thrombosis, or to those taking MAO inhibitors.

- Administer with caution to clients with diabetes, thyroid disorders, arrhythmias, hypertension, sulfite sensitivity, or severe cardiac disease.

- Monitor blood pressure during therapy.

- Assess for extravasation because this drug may cause necrosis of tissue at injection sites; administer phentolamine if extravasation occurs.

Generic: normal serum albumin (NOR-mal SEE-rum AL-byoo-min)

Brand: Albuminar, Plasbumin

Classification(s): Plasma volume expander; plasma derivative

Generic: nortriptyline (nor-TRIP-till-een)

Brand: Pamelor

Classification(s): Antidepressant, tricyclic

Side Effects: Allergic reactions, fever, chills, rash, shortness of breath

Nursing Implications and Precautions:

- Do not administer to clients with severe anemia or cardiac failure.

- Monitor vital signs during the infusion to examine for too-rapid increases in blood pressure; adjust flow rate as necessary.

- Monitor the injection site for extravasation.

- Discard any colored solutions or those with turbidity.

- Administer concentrated solutions with caution to clients with low cardiac reserve because rapid changes in blood pressure or pulmonary edema may result.

- If diluting the drug, use 5% dextrose or normal saline.

Side Effects: Suicidal ideation, dry mouth, sedation, confusion, orthostatic hypotension, urinary retention, tachycardia, drowsiness, blurred vision, constipation, neuroleptic malignant syndrome (rare)

Nursing Implications and Precautions:

- Monitor for worsening depression and suicidal ideation.

- Advise client to avoid driving and other hazardous activities until the effects of the drug are known.

- Advise client to continue taking the drug, even if symptoms resolve.

- Advise client that the drug must be taken several weeks before the full effects of the drug are noticed.

- Use with caution in clients with benign prostatic hyperplasia, hepatic impairment, hyperthyroidism, and Parkinson's disease.

- Advise client to move slowly from a lying to a standing position to prevent light-headedness.

- Do not administer this drug to clients taking monoamine oxidase (MAO) inhibitors.

Generic: olanzaprine (oh-LAN-zah-preen)

Brand: Zyprexa

Classification(s): Antipsychotic, atypical; antimanic

Side Effects: Weight gain, constipation, drowsiness, dizziness, dry mouth, unusual changes in behavior, neuroleptic malignant syndrome (rare), orthostatic hypotension, akathisia

Nursing Implications and Precautions:

- Monitor regularly for weight gain, hyperglycemia, and hyperlipidemia.

- Use with caution in older adult clients with dementia-related psychoses because there is an increased risk of death.

- Monitor for unusual changes in behavior, worsening depression, and suicidal ideation.

- Use with caution in clients with diabetes or seizure disorders.

- Advise client to avoid driving and other hazardous activities until the effects of the drug are known.

- Assess for tardive dyskinesia; discontinue drug and notify prescriber immediately.

- Advise client to move slowly from a lying to a standing position to prevent light-headedness.

- Advise client to take drug for the entire length of time prescribed, even if feeling better.

- Advise client to limit or eliminate alcohol use during therapy because this may cause excessive drowsiness.

Generic: **olmesartan** (OLE-meh-SAR-tan)

Brand: Benicar

Classification(s): Antihypertensive; angiotensin II receptor antagonist

Generic: **olopatadine ophthalmic drops**
(OH-low-PAT-ah-deen)

Brand: Patanol

Classification(s): Ocular antihistamine

Side Effects: Diarrhea, dyspepsia, fatigue, rhabdomyolysis (rare), fetal death and injury

Nursing Implications and Precautions:

- Instruct women of childbearing age to use effective birth control method (pregnancy Category D in second and third trimesters).
- Advise the female client to immediately notify the prescriber of known or suspected pregnancy.
- Monitor blood pressure during therapy to evaluate drug effectiveness.
- Advise client to take drug for the entire length of time prescribed, even if feeling better.
- Assess electrolytes and correct salt or volume depletion prior to starting therapy.
- Administer with caution to clients with renal impairment, heart failure, or renal artery stenosis.
- Advise client not to use salt substitutes containing potassium, unless directed by the prescriber.
- Monitor for myopathy and discontinue drug if symptoms of muscle pain or weakness persist.

Side Effects: Headache, blurred vision, burning/stinging, dry eye, foreign body sensation, hyperemia, keratitis, eyelid edema, asthenia, cold syndrome, pharyngitis, rhinitis, sinusitis, changes in taste

Nursing Implications and Precautions:

- Advise client to not exceed the prescribed dose because this may reduce the drug's effectiveness.
- Advise client to remove contact lenses before using the drug and to wait at least 10 minutes before reinsertion.
- Advise client to wait at least 5 minutes between applications of other topical ophthalmic drugs.
- Teach client proper method of instilling drug on the eye.
- Advise client not to use any other eye drops unless approved by the prescriber.

Generic: omeprazole (oh-MEP-rah-zole)

Brand: Prilosec

Classification(s): Antiulcer; proton pump inhibitor

Side Effects: Headache, diarrhea, abdominal pain, nausea, flatulence, constipation

Nursing Implications and Precautions:

- Administer with caution with drugs for which gastric pH affects bioavailability (such as ketoconazole, iron salts, and digoxin).

- Administer drug at least 1 hour before a meal.

- Advise clients taking extended-release forms to swallow the drug whole and not to crush, split, or chew the capsules.

- Advise client to continue taking the drug for the entire length of time prescribed, even if feeling better.

- Advise client to notify the prescriber if symptoms have not resolved following 4–8 weeks of therapy.

- Do not administer concurrently with atazanavir or nelfinavir.

- Monitor concurrent therapy with drugs metabolized by cytochrome P450 (such as warfarin, phenytoin, cyclosporine, and benzodiazepines) because omeprazole can prolong their elimination.

Generic: **oxycodone** (OX-ee-KOH-doan)

Brand: OxyContin, others

Classification(s): Narcotic (opiate agonist) analgesic

Side Effects: Respiratory depression, light-headedness, sedation, nausea and vomiting, dysphoria, constipation

Nursing Implications and Precautions:

- Advise client to store drug in a safe place, away from children or those who may take the drug for recreational purposes.

- Monitor carefully in clients with high potential for substance abuse.

- Do not administer to clients with head injury or high intracranial pressure.

- Monitor for interactions with other CNS depressants.

- Monitor for excessive sedation.

- Advise client to avoid driving and other hazardous activities until the effects of the drug are known.

- Advise client to limit or eliminate alcohol use during therapy because this may cause excessive drowsiness.

- Do not administer to clients with paralytic ileus, acute or severe asthma, or severe respiratory depression.

- Advise client to not discontinue the drug abruptly.

- Do not administer extended-release forms to clients unless they are opioid tolerant.

Generic: **oxybutynin** (OX-ee-BYOO-tye-nin)

Brand: Ditropan

Classification(s): Genitourinary antispasmodic; anticholinergic; antimuscarinic

Generic: **oxymetazoline** (OX-ee-me-TAZ-oh-leen)

Brand: Afrin

Classification(s): Decongestant; nasal preparation

Side Effects: Anticholinergic effects (dry mouth, dizziness, blurred vision, constipation, nausea), drowsiness

Nursing Implications and Precautions:

- Do not administer to clients with uncontrolled glaucoma, gastrointestinal obstruction, paralytic ileus, intestinal atony, severe colitis, myasthenia gravis, megacolon, obstructive uropathies, and unstable cardiovascular status in acute hemorrhage.

- Administer with caution to clients with diarrhea, hepatic or renal impairment, autonomic neuropathy, hyperthyroidism, cardiovascular disease, hiatal hernia, or under conditions of exposure to extreme heat.

- Advise client to avoid driving and other hazardous activities until the effects of the drug are known.

- Advise client to limit or eliminate alcohol use during therapy because this may cause excessive drowsiness.

- Advise client to notify health care providers of all medications taken because oxybutynin interacts with multiple drugs.

- Advise client to avoid high environmental temperatures or heavy exercise during therapy because heat stroke may occur.

Side Effects: Palpitations, sneezing and nasal burning, stinging, dryness, irritation

Nursing Implications and Precautions:

- Administer with caution to clients with hypertension, glaucoma, hyperthyroidism, diabetes, heart disease, or urinary retention.

- Advise client to take drug exactly as prescribed and not use larger doses without consulting with the prescriber.

- Advise client to limit use of the drug to 3–5 days because longer use can cause rebound congestion and damage the nasal mucosa.

- Advise client to clear the nose before administering the drug.

Generic: **pantoprazole** (pan-TOH-prah-zole)

Brand: Protonix

Classification(s): Antiulcer; gastric proton pump inhibitor; antisecretory

Side Effects: Headache, diarrhea, abdominal pain, nausea, flatulence, arthralgia, dry mouth

Nursing Implications and Precautions:

- Administer with caution with drugs for which gastric pH affects bioavailability (such as ketoconazole, iron salts, and digoxin).
- Administer drug at least 1 hour before a meal.
- Advise clients taking extended-release forms to swallow the drug whole and not to crush, split, or chew the capsules.
- Advise client to continue taking the drug for the entire length of time prescribed, even if feeling better.
- Advise client to notify the prescriber if symptoms have not resolved following 4–8 weeks of therapy.
- Do not administer concurrently with atazanavir or nelfinavir.

Generic: **paroxetine** (par-OX-ah-teen)

Brand: Paxil

Classification(s): Antidepressant; antianxiety; selective serotonin 5-HT reuptake inhibitor (SSRI)

Side Effects: Suicidal ideation, insomnia, anorexia, nausea, vomiting, sexual disorders, drowsiness, abnormal bleeding, sweating, tremor, serotonin syndrome and neuroleptic malignant syndrome (rare), fetal injury and death (pregnancy Category D)

Nursing Implications and Precautions:

- Do not administer to clients with suicidal ideation.
- Monitor for worsening depression and suicidal ideation.
- Advise client to avoid driving and other hazardous activities until the effects of the drug are known.
- Advise client to continue taking the drug, even if feeling better.
- Advise client that the drug must be taken several weeks before the full effects of the drug are noticed.
- Monitor for unusual bruising or bleeding.
- Advise client to not take aspirin or other drugs that affect coagulation unless directed by the prescriber.

- Do not administer this drug to clients taking monoamine oxidase (MAO) inhibitors.
- Advise client to limit or eliminate alcohol use during therapy because this may cause excessive drowsiness.
- Advise client to report changes in sexual performance, including ejaculatory delay, decreased libido, and anorgasmia.
- Monitor for weight gain or loss during therapy.
- Advise women of childbearing age to use effective birth control method and to immediately notify the prescriber of known or suspected pregnancy.

Generic: penicillin VK (pen-uh-SILL-in)

Brand: Pen-Vee K, Veetids

Classification(s): Beta-lactam antibiotic

Generic: phenazopyridine (FEN-az-oh-PEER-ih-deen)

Brand: Pyridium

Classification(s): Urinary tract analgesic

Side Effects: Nausea/vomiting, diarrhea, urticaria, allergic reactions

Nursing Implications and Precautions:

- Assess for history of hypersensitivity to penicillins or other antibiotics.

- Advise client to take drug for the entire length of time prescribed, even if symptoms of infection have resolved.

- Monitor for allergic reactions, including anaphylaxis.

- Administer drug on an empty stomach.

- Monitor for pseudomembranous colitis (severe diarrhea).

Side Effects: Headache, rash, GI upset, methemoglobinemia, hemolytic anemia, nephrotoxicity, hepatotoxicity

Nursing Implications and Precautions:

- Do not administer to clients with renal insufficiency.

- Monitor for hepatic impairment: Yellow discoloration of skin or sclera may indicate poor renal excretion.

- Advise client that the drug may permanently stain contact lenses.

- Monitor for anemia.

- Advise client that the drug causes a harmless red-orange discoloration of the urine.

- Advise client to take drug exactly as prescribed.

Generic: phenobarbital (FEE-no-BAR-bih-tall)

Brand: Luminal

Classification(s): Anticonvulsant; sedative-hypnotic; barbiturate

Side Effects: Sedation; headache; hangover effect; hallucinations; blood dyscrasias; nausea/vomiting; deficiencies in folic acid, vitamin D, and calcium; paradoxical CNS stimulation

Nursing Implications and Precautions:

- Advise client to avoid driving and other hazardous activities until the effects of the drug are known.

- Advise client to continue taking the drug, even if feeling better.

- Advise client to limit or eliminate alcohol use during therapy because this may cause excessive drowsiness.

- Assess for signs of overdose or abuse (confusion, sedation, slurred speech, coma).

- Administer with caution concurrently with other CNS depressants because excessive sedation may result.

- Do not administer to clients with history of drug abuse or suicidal ideation.

- Advise client to not discontinue the drug abruptly because this will cause seizures and other withdrawal symptoms.

- Advise client to take the drug immediately prior to expected sleep.

- Advise client to store drug in a safe place, away from children.

Generic: phentermine (FEN-tare-meen)

Brand: Adipex-P, ProFast SA

Classification(s): Appetite suppressant; anorexiant

Side Effects: CNS stimulation, dizziness, palpitations, arrhythmias, hypertension, psychosis, dry mouth, GI disturbances, urticaria, impotence, primary pulmonary hypertension

Nursing Implications and Precautions:

- Do not administer to clients with arteriosclerosis, cardiovascular disease, hyperthyroidism, glaucoma, agitation, or history of drug or alcohol abuse.

- Do not administer this drug within 2 weeks of taking monoamine oxidase (MAO) inhibitors.

- Administer with caution to clients with hypertension and diabetes.

- Monitor for dyspnea, angina pectoris, syncope, lower extremity edema, or other symptoms of primary pulmonary hypertension and discontinue drug if these occur.

- Advise client not to take this drug longer than a few weeks because tolerance to the anorectic effect occurs.

- Advise client that use with alcohol may increase the potential for side effects.

- Advise client to not take drug with any other diet products without notifying the prescriber.

- Advise client to store drug in a safe place, away from children or those who may take the drug for recreational purposes.

- Advise client to not discontinue the drug abruptly.

Generic: phenytoin (FEN-ih-tow-in)

Brand: Dilantin

Classification(s): Anticonvulsant; hydantoin

Side Effects: Nystagmus, ataxia, slurred speech, decreased coordination, dizziness, confusion, nausea/vomiting, gingival hyperplasia, Stevens-Johnson syndrome (rare), fetal toxicity

Nursing Implications and Precautions:

- Administer with caution to clients with diabetes, liver impairment, and porphyria.

- Advise client to not discontinue the drug abruptly because serious seizures may result.

- Monitor for rash and discontinue drug if this occurs.

- Monitor serum levels: 10–20 mcg/mL is considered the therapeutic range.

- Advise client to regularly visit dental health professionals and maintain good oral hygiene.

- Advise the female client to immediately notify the prescriber of known or suspected pregnancy.

- Advise client to limit or eliminate alcohol use during therapy because alcohol use will increase the side effects of the drug.

- Advise client to notify health care providers of all medications taken because phenytoin interacts with multiple drugs.

- Monitor for behavioral changes and suicidal ideation.

- Monitor blood glucose levels in diabetic clients because this drug may cause hyperglycemia.

- Advise client to continue taking the drug, even if symptoms resolve.

Generic: pioglitazone (PYE-oh-GLIT-ag-zone)

Brand: Actos

Classification(s): Antidiabetic; insulin sensitizer; thiazolidinedione

Side Effects: Upper respiratory infection, headache, sinusitis, pharyngitis, myalgia, edema, weight gain, hypoglycemia, changes in serum lipids, risk of fracture (women)

Nursing Implications and Precautions:

- Do not administer to clients with Class III or IV heart failure.

- Administer with caution to clients with Class II heart failure, edema, or liver impairment.

- Monitor for symptoms of heart failure and discontinue drug if these occur.

- Assess baseline liver function and do not start therapy if ALT is greater than two and one-half time the upper limits of normal.

- Monitor hepatic enzymes regularly during therapy.

- Advise client that resumption of menstruation may occur and this may result in unintended pregnancy; contraception should be recommended.

- Assess for edema and weight gain during therapy because these may indicate impending heart failure.

- Monitor serum glucose and assess for hypoglycemia during therapy.

- Advise client of the importance of adhering to all exercise, weight control, and dietary instructions provided by the prescriber.

- Advise client to monitor serum glucose levels more frequently during infections or periods of stress or heavy exercise.

Generic: **polyethylene glycol (oral)** (pol-ee-ETH-ill-een GLY-kol)

Brand: MiraLax, Glycolax

Classification(s): Laxative

Generic: **potassium chloride** (poe-TASS-ee-um KLOR-ide)

Brand: K-Dur, Klor-Con, Micro-K

Classification(s): Electrolyte replacement solution

Side Effects: Loose, watery, frequent stools

Nursing Implications and Precautions:

- Do not administer to clients with known or suspected bowel obstruction.
- Administer with caution to clients with renal impairment, nausea/vomiting, abdominal pain, bulimia, or irritable bowel syndrome.
- Advise client not to use this drug more than once per day, or for more than 7 days.
- If severe diarrhea or bloody stools occur, discontinue drug.

Side Effects: Hyperkalemia, nausea/vomiting, flatulence, diarrhea, esophageal and GI ulceration, bleeding, obstruction, perforation

Nursing Implications and Precautions:

- Do not administer to clients with hyperkalemia, chronic renal disease, acute dehydration, heat cramps, adrenal insufficiency, acidosis, alkalosis, esophageal compression due to enlarged left atrium, or decreased GI motility.
- Administer with caution to clients with renal or cardiac disease.
- Assess for GI bleeding or ulceration, and discontinue drug if these occur.
- Monitor serum potassium level, acid-base balance, and ECG during therapy.
- Administer with caution concurrently with potassium-sparing diuretics.
- Advise client taking extended-release forms to swallow the drug whole and not to crush, split, or chew the tablets or capsules.

Generic: pravastatin (pray-vah-STAT-in)

Brand: Pravachol

Classification(s): Antilipemic; statin; HMG-CoA reductase inhibitor

Side Effects: Headache, intestinal cramping, dizziness, elevated serum transaminases, myopathy, fetal toxicity

Nursing Implications and Precautions:

- Assess baseline liver enzymes before starting therapy and monitor during therapy for possible hepatotoxicity.

- Do not administer to clients with active liver disease or who are pregnant.

- Assess for myopathy (muscle pain and weakness).

- Instruct women of childbearing age to use effective birth control method (pregnancy Category X).

- Advise client to continue taking the drug, even if feeling fine.

- Administer drug at least 1 hour before or at least 4 hours after taking bile acid-binding resins such as cholestyramine or colestipol.

- Advise clients taking extended-release forms to swallow the drug whole and not to crush, split, or chew the capsules.

- Advise client to limit or eliminate alcohol use during therapy because this increases the risk for hepatic toxicity.

Generic: prednisone (PRED-niss-ohn)

Brand: Deltasone, Sterapred

Classification(s): Immunosuppressant; anti-inflammatory; adrenal corticosteroid

Side Effects: Adrenal insufficiency/atrophy, Cushing's syndrome, masking of active infection, glaucoma, cataracts, secondary infections, electrolyte deficiencies, hypertension, behavioral changes, osteoporosis, peptic ulcer, dermal atrophy, carbohydrate intolerance

Nursing Implications and Precautions:

- Do not administer to clients with systemic mycoses or other severe infections.
- Do not administer immunizations with live vaccines during therapy.
- Administer with caution to clients with any viral, bacterial, fungal, or protozoal infection.
- Administer with caution to clients with hypothyroidism, hepatic cirrhosis, renal insufficiency, peptic ulcer, hypertension, osteoporosis, or diabetes.
- Advise client to take drug exactly as prescribed and not to discontinue the drug or change the dose without consulting with the prescriber.

- Monitor weight, growth, and fluid and electrolyte balance.
- Monitor blood pressure during prolonged therapy.
- Advise client to notify prescriber of any unusual stress, serious illness, fever, or infection because doses may need to be increased during these periods.
- Advise clients to avoid crowds or places where they may be exposed to people with infections.

Generic: pregabalin (pre-GAB-ah-lin)

Brand: Lyrica

Classification(s): Anticonvulsant; analgesic; antianxiety; GABA analog

Side Effects: Somnolence, dizziness, ataxia, angioedema, visual disturbances, weight gain, peripheral edema, asthenia, confusion, dry mouth

Nursing Implications and Precautions:

- Advise client to continue taking the drug, even if feeling better.
- Advise client to not discontinue the drug abruptly because this may cause seizures.
- Assess for myopathy and discontinue drug if markedly elevated creatine kinase (CK) levels occur.
- Administer with caution to clients with heart failure, ocular conditions, or suicidal ideation.
- Monitor for suicidal ideation.
- Advise client to limit or eliminate alcohol use during therapy because this increases drowsiness.
- Monitor for angioedema and discontinue drug immediately if this occurs.
- Advise client to avoid driving and other hazardous activities until the effects of the drug are known.
- Monitor carefully in clients with a potential for substance abuse.

Generic: promethazine (pro-METH-ah-zeen)

Brand: Phenergan

Classification(s): Antihistamine; antiemetic; antivertigo

Side Effects: Drowsiness, lowered seizure threshold, cholestatic jaundice, anticholinergic effects (dry mouth, dizziness, blurred vision, nausea), extrapyramidal effects, photosensitivity, hypo- or hypertension, rash, blood dyscrasias, nausea, neonatal platelet abnormalities, respiratory depression (children)

Nursing Implications and Precautions:

- Do not administer to clients with history of sleep apnea, asthma and lower respiratory disorders, uncomplicated nausea in children, dehydrated or ill children (especially Reye's syndrome), and to children under 2 years of age.

- Monitor for respiratory depression, especially in children.

- Do not administer this drug to clients taking monoamine oxidase (MAO) inhibitors.

- Administer with caution to clients with glaucoma, hepatic impairment, seizure disorders, cardiovascular disease, bone marrow suppression, or gastrointestinal (GI) or urinary obstruction.

- If taken for motion sickness, administer 30–60 minutes before expected travel.

- Advise client to limit or eliminate alcohol use during therapy because this may cause excessive drowsiness.

Generic: propoxyphene with acetaminophin (APAP)
(pro-POX-ee-feen ah-seet-ah-MIN-oh-fen)

Brand: Darvocet-N

Classification(s): Narcotic analgesic; opiate agonist

Generic: propranolol (proh-PRAN-oh-lole)

Brand: Inderal

Classification(s): Antihypertensive; antiarrhythmic, class II; antianginal; beta-adrenergic receptor antagonist

Side Effects: Respiratory depression, light-headedness, sedation, nausea/vomiting, dysphoria, constipation

Nursing Implications and Precautions:

- Do not administer to clients with paralytic ileus, severe asthma, or severe respiratory depression or to those with high potential for substance abuse.
- Monitor for interactions with other CNS depressants.
- Monitor for excessive sedation.
- Advise client to avoid driving and other hazardous activities until the effects of the drug are known.
- Advise client to limit or eliminate alcohol use during therapy because this may cause excessive drowsiness.
- With high doses of acetaminophen, monitor for hepatotoxicity.
- Assess for signs of overdose or abuse (confusion, sedation, slurred speech, coma).
- Advise client to store drug in a safe place, away from children or those who may take the drug for recreational purposes.
- Monitor for suicidal ideation.
- Advise client not to take over-the-counter medications containing acetaminophen.

Side Effects: Nausea, vomiting, diarrhea, bradycardia, hypotension, fatigue, dizziness, diarrhea, insomnia, hyperglycemia

Nursing Implications and Precautions:

- Do not administer to clients with severe bradycardia, heart block greater than first degree, cardiogenic shock, or decompensated heart failure.
- Monitor for worsening heart failure or fluid retention.
- Advise client to not discontinue the drug abruptly because this may precipitate angina pain or myocardial infarction.
- Monitor blood glucose levels in clients with diabetes.
- Administer with caution to clients with diabetes, severe hepatic impairment, hyperthyroidism, or asthma.
- Advise client to move slowly from a lying to a standing position to prevent light-headedness.

Generic: pseudoephedrine (SUE-doe-ee-FED-rin)

Brand: Sudafed

Classification(s): Nasal decongestant; alpha- and beta-adrenergic receptor agonist

Generic: quetiapine (kwe-TYE-ah-peen)

Brand: Seroquel

Classification(s): Antipsychotic, atypical

Side Effects: Nervousness, dizziness, palpitations, insomnia

Nursing Implications and Precautions:

- Do not administer this drug within 2 weeks of taking monoamine oxidase (MAO) inhibitors.

- Administer with caution to clients with asthma, glaucoma, hyperthyroidism, hypertension, cardiovascular disease, or gastrointestinal (GI) or urinary obstruction.

- Advise client not to take this drug for more than 7 days, unless directed by the prescriber.

- Advise client that over-the-counter forms are not recommended for children under 12 years of age.

- Advise client not to crush or chew the extended-release tablets.

Side Effects: Weight gain, constipation, drowsiness, malaise, dizziness, dry mouth, abdominal pain, neuroleptic malignant syndrome (rare), orthostatic hypotension, asthenia

Nursing Implications and Precautions:

- Monitor regularly for weight gain, hyperglycemia, and hyperlipidemia.

- Use with caution in older adult clients with dementia-related psychoses because there is an increased risk of death.

- Monitor for suicidal ideation.

- Advise client to avoid driving and other hazardous activities until the effects of the drug are known.

- Assess for tardive dyskinesia; discontinue drug and notify prescriber immediately.

- Advise client to move slowly from a lying to a standing position to prevent light-headedness.

- Advise client to take drug for the entire length of time prescribed, even if feeling better.

- Advise client to limit or eliminate alcohol use during therapy because this may cause excessive drowsiness.

- Monitor for cataract development.

Generic: quinapril (KWIN-ah-prill)

Brand: Accupril

Classification(s): Antihypertensive; angiotensin-converting enzyme (ACE) inhibitor

Generic: rabeprazole (rah-BEP-rah-zole)

Brand: Aciphex

Classification(s): Antiulcer; proton pump inhibitor

Side Effects: Headache, cough, dizziness, orthostatic hypotension, angioedema, hyperkalemia, fetal death and injury

Nursing Implications and Precautions:

- Instruct women of childbearing age to use effective birth control method (pregnancy Category D).
- Advise the female client to immediately notify the prescriber of known or suspected pregnancy.
- Use with caution in clients with kidney or liver disease.
- Advise client to limit or eliminate alcohol use during therapy.
- Monitor blood pressure during therapy to evaluate drug effectiveness.
- Advise client to move slowly from a lying to a standing position to prevent light-headedness.
- Advise client to drink at least 6–8 glasses of water each day.
- Advise client to take drug for the entire length of time prescribed.
- Advise client not to use salt substitutes containing potassium, unless directed by the prescriber.

Side Effects: Headache, diarrhea, abdominal pain, nausea, constipation

Nursing Implications and Precautions:

- Administer with caution to clients with severe hepatic impairment.
- Administer with caution with drugs for which gastric pH affects bioavailability (such as ketoconazole, iron salts, and digoxin).
- Administer drug at least 1 hour before a meal.
- Advise clients taking extended-release forms to swallow the drug whole and not to crush, split, or chew the capsules.
- Advise client to continue taking the drug for the entire length of time prescribed, even if feeling better.
- Advise client to notify the prescriber if symptoms have not resolved following 4–8 weeks of therapy.
- Do not administer concurrently with atazanavir.

Generic: **raloxifene** (rah-LOX-ih-feen)

Brand: Evista

Classification(s): Osteoporosis prophylactic; selective estrogen receptor antagonist/agonist

Side Effects: Hot flashes, leg cramps, peripheral edema, flu syndrome, arthralgia, sweating; venous thromboembolic events, fetal toxicity (pregnancy Category X).

Nursing Implications and Precautions:

- Obtain serum lipid and calcium levels and bone density measurements prior to and during therapy to assess drug effectiveness.

- Do not administer to clients with history of venous thromboembolic events, or to women who are nursing or pregnant; not for use in premenopausal women.

- Administer with caution to clients with concomitant systemic estrogen therapy, coronary heart disease, or risk of coronary event, hepatic, or renal impairment.

- Discontinue drug at least 72 hours before, and during prolonged immobilization; resume when fully ambulatory.

- If client is concurrently taking warfarin, monitor prothrombin time regularly.

- Prior to starting therapy, rule out pregnancy in women of childbearing potential and advise these clients to use effective contraception during therapy.

- Advise client to avoid sitting still for long periods of time during travel.

- Advise client to immediately report symptoms of thromboembolic disease during therapy (chest pain, shortness of breath, pain in calves).

Generic: ramipril (RAM-ah-prill)

Brand: Altace

Classification(s): Antihypertensive; angiotensin-converting enzyme (ACE) inhibitor

Generic: ranitidine (rah-NIT-ih-deen)

Brand: Zantac

Classification(s): Antiulcer; antisecretory (H2-receptor antagonist)

Side Effects

Side Effects: Headache, cough, dizziness, orthostatic hypotension, angioedema, hyperkalemia, fetal death and injury

Nursing Implications and Precautions:

- Instruct women of childbearing age to use effective birth control method (pregnancy Category D).
- Advise the female client to immediately notify the prescriber of known or suspected pregnancy.
- Use with caution in clients with kidney or liver disease.
- Advise client to limit or eliminate alcohol use during therapy.
- Monitor blood pressure during therapy to evaluate drug effectiveness.
- Advise client to move slowly from a lying to a standing position to prevent light-headedness.
- Advise client to drink at least 6–8 glasses of water each day.
- Advise client to take drug for the entire length of time prescribed.
- Advise client not to use salt substitutes containing potassium, unless directed by the prescriber.

Side Effects: Headache, dizziness, constipation, diarrhea, pneumonia

Nursing Implications and Precautions:

- Do not administer to clients with acute porphyria.
- Administer with caution to clients with hepatic or renal impairment. Advise client to notify the prescriber if symptoms have not resolved in 4–6 weeks.
- Advise client to take drug for the entire length of time prescribed, even if symptoms have resolved.
- Administer drug 15–60 minutes before eating food or drinks that cause heartburn.
- Advise client to limit alcohol use during therapy.
- Advise client to immediately report symptoms of pneumonia (chest pain, fever, fatigue, shortness of breath).
- Advise client to dissolve the effervescent tablets and granules in 6–8 ounces of water before drinking.

Generic: reteplase (REH-teh-place)

Brand: Activase

Classification(s): Thrombolytic; tissue plasminogen activator (t-PA)

Generic: risedronate (ris-ED-roh-nate)

Brand: Actonel

Classification(s): Bone resorption inhibitor; osteoporosis treatment; bisphosphonate

Side Effects: Bleeding, including intracranial hemorrhage and at external and internal sites

Nursing Implications and Precautions:

- Do not administer drug to clients with history of cerebrovascular accident, intracranial or intraspinal surgery or trauma, active internal bleeding, intracranial neoplasm, arteriovenous malformation or aneurysm, uncontrolled hypertension, and bleeding diathesis.

- Avoid intramuscular injections and nonessential handling of client during treatment because these increase the risk of bleeding.

- Monitor for bleeding, which may occur at any internal or external site; discontinue if serious bleeding occurs.

- Monitor for extravasation.

- Monitor for excessive bleeding in clients concurrently taking anticoagulant or antiplatelet drugs.

- Monitor vital signs frequently during therapy.

Side Effects: Diarrhea, constipation, flatulence, nausea, vomiting, headache, metallic taste, musculoskeletal pain, pathologic fractures, osteonecrosis of the jaw

Nursing Implications and Precautions:

- Administer drug with plain water, preferably 1–2 hours before breakfast.

- Ensure that client remains upright for at least 30 minutes after taking drug.

- Advise client to immediately report jaw pain, swelling, loose teeth, or gum infections.

- Do not administer with medicines that contain calcium, aluminum, or magnesium.

- Assess results of periodic bone mineral density tests to ensure effectiveness of therapy.

- Advise client to include adequate amounts of vitamin D and calcium in the diet.

Generic: risperidone (ris-PER-ih-doan)

Brand: Risperdal

Classification(s): Antipsychotic, atypical

Side Effects: Increased appetite, constipation, drowsiness, fatigue, dizziness, dry mouth, agitation, neuroleptic malignant syndrome (rare), orthostatic hypotension, akathisia, stroke, upper respiratory tract infection, abdominal pain, dyspepsia

Nursing Implications and Precautions:

- Monitor regularly for hyperglycemia.
- Use with caution in older adult clients with dementia-related psychoses because there is an increased risk of death.
- Monitor for suicidal ideation.
- Use with caution in clients with diabetes or seizure disorders.
- Advise client to avoid driving and other hazardous activities until the effects of the drug are known.
- Assess for tardive dyskinesia; discontinue drug and notify prescriber immediately.
- Advise client to move slowly from a lying to a standing position to prevent light-headedness.
- Advise client to take drug for the entire length of time prescribed, even if feeling better.
- Advise client to limit or eliminate alcohol use during therapy because this may cause excessive drowsiness.

Generic: ropinirole (roe-PIN-ih-role)

Brand: Requip

Classification(s): Antiparkinson; dopamine receptor agonist

Side Effects: Somnolence (including sudden sleep onset), postural hypotension, nausea/vomiting, abdominal pain/discomfort, dizziness, headache, hallucinations

Nursing Implications and Precautions:

- Monitor for daytime sleepiness or sudden onset of sleep during daily activities.

- Advise client to move slowly from a lying to a standing position to prevent light-headedness.

- Administer with caution to clients with dyskinesia, sleep disorders, severe renal or hepatic impairment, severe cardiovascular disease, hypertension, or psychotic disorders.

- Advise client to not discontinue the drug abruptly.

- Monitor for hallucinations, especially in older adult clients.

- Advise client to discontinue smoking because this reduces the effectiveness of the drug.

- Advise client to limit or eliminate alcohol use during therapy because this may cause excessive drowsiness.

Generic: rosiglitazone (ro-zee-GLIT-ah-zone)

Brand: Avandia

Classification(s): Antihyperglycemic

Side Effects: Upper respiratory infection, headache, myalgia, edema, weight gain, hypoglycemia, macular edema, myocardial ischemia, changes in serum lipids, risk of fracture (women)

Nursing Implications and Precautions:

- Do not administer to clients with Class III or IV heart failure.

- Administer with caution to clients with Class II heart failure, edema, or liver impairment.

- Monitor for symptoms of heart failure and discontinue drug if these occur.

- Assess baseline liver function and do not start therapy if ALT is greater than two and one-half times the upper limit of normal.

- Monitor hepatic enzymes regularly during therapy.

- Advise client that resumption of menstruation may occur and this may result in unintended pregnancy; contraception should be recommended.

- Assess for edema and weight gain during therapy because these may indicate impending heart failure.

- Monitor serum glucose and assess for hypoglycemia during therapy.

- Advise client of the importance of adhering to all exercise, weight control, and dietary instructions provided by the prescriber.

- Advise client to monitor serum glucose levels more frequently during infections or periods of stress or heavy exercise.

Generic: rosuvastatin (row-SUE-vah-STAH-tin)

Brand: Crestor

Classification(s): Antihyperlipemic; HMG-CoA reductase inhibitor (statin)

Side Effects: Intestinal cramping, asthenia, headache, arthralgia, myopathy, fetal toxicity (pregnancy Category X)

Nursing Implications and Precautions:

- Do not administer to clients with active liver disease, unexplained persistent elevations in serum transaminases, or to nursing or pregnant women.

- Monitor liver enzymes during therapy for possible hepatotoxicity.

- Assess for myopathy (muscle pain and weakness) and discontinue drug if this occurs.

- Advise client to immediately report unexplained skeletal muscle pain or weakness.

- Administer with caution concurrently with strong CYP3A4 enzyme inhibitors (such as clarithromycin, azole antifungals, grapefruit juice, or cyclosporine).

- Instruct women of childbearing age to use effective birth control method.

- Advise client to continue taking the drug, even if feeling fine.

- Advise client to limit or eliminate alcohol use during therapy because this increases the risk for hepatic toxicity.

- If concurrently taking warfarin, monitor INR regularly because rosuvastatin prolongs INR.

Generic: **salmeterol** (sal-MET-terr-oll)

Brand: Serevent

Classification(s): Bronchodilator; beta$_2$-adrenergic agonist; respiratory smooth muscle relaxant

Side Effects: Paradoxical bronchospasm, increased blood pressure, tachycardia, ECG changes, allergic reactions, nervousness, increased risk of asthma-related death

Nursing Implications and Precautions:

- Administer with caution to clients with cardiovascular disorders such as coronary artery disease, dysrhythmias, or hypertension.

- If using an inhaler, teach client proper use of the device.

- Do not administer with a beta-adrenergic blocker, unless directed by the prescriber.

- If administering with a diuretic, monitor for potential hypokalemia.

- Advise client to notify the prescriber immediately if the drug stops working well or if more doses per day are needed to prevent breathing difficulties.

- Monitor carefully for signs of worsening asthma because salmeterol (and other long-acting beta agonists) may increase the risk of asthma-related death.

- Do not administer with other long-acting beta agonists unless directed by the prescriber.

- Advise client that this drug should not be used to treat an acute asthma attack that has already begun.

- Advise client to continue taking this drug, even if feeling better.

Generic: sertraline (SERR-trah-leen)

Brand: Zoloft

Classification(s): Antidepressant; selective serotonin reuptake inhibitor (SSRI)

Side Effects: Suicidal ideation, insomnia, fatigue, dry mouth, tremor, sexual disorders, drowsiness, abnormal bleeding, sweating, serotonin syndrome and neuroleptic malignant syndrome (rare)

Nursing Implications and Precautions:

- Do not administer to clients with suicidal ideation.
- Monitor for worsening depression and suicidal ideation.
- Advise client to avoid driving and other hazardous activities until the effects of the drug are known.
- Advise client to continue taking the drug, even if feeling better.
- Advise client that the drug must be taken several weeks before the full effects of the drug are noticed.
- Monitor for unusual bruising or bleeding.
- Advise client to not take aspirin or other drugs that affect coagulation unless directed by the prescriber.
- Do not administer this drug to clients taking monoamine oxidase (MAO) inhibitors.
- Advise client to limit or eliminate alcohol use during therapy because this may cause excessive drowsiness.
- Advise client to report changes in sexual performance, including ejaculatory delay, decreased libido, and anorgasmia.

Generic: sildenafil (sil-DEN-ah-fill)

Brand: Viagra

Classification(s): Pulmonary antihypertensive; phosphodiesterase (PDE) inhibitor; pulmonary antihypertensive

Side Effects: Headache, flushing, dyspepsia, nasal congestion, visual disturbances, priapism

Nursing Implications and Precautions:

- Do not administer this drug to clients concurrently taking organic nitrates or sodium nitroprusside.

- Administer with caution to clients with myocardial infarction, stroke, or life-threatening arrhythmia within 6 months; blood pressure less than 90/50 mmHg or greater than 170/110 mmHg; unstable angina; left ventricular outflow obstruction; anatomical penile deformation; predisposition to priapism; bleeding disorders; active peptic ulcer; or retinitis pigmentosa.

- Monitor blood pressure during therapy in clients concurrently taking antihypertensives because the sildenafil may significantly lower blood pressure.

- Advise client to promptly seek medical attention if the drug causes a sudden loss of vision or hearing or if a painful erection lasts longer than 4 hours.

- Advise client not to share the medication.

- Advise client to take drug exactly as prescribed and not to take it more frequently.

- Advise client to take the drug 30–60 minutes prior to expected sexual activity.

Generic: **simvastatin** (SIM-vah-stah-tin)

Brand: Zocor

Classification(s): Antihyperlipemic; HMG-CoA reductase inhibitor (statin)

Side Effects: Upper respiratory infection, abdominal pain, headache, myopathy, fetal toxicity (pregnancy Category X)

Nursing Implications and Precautions:

- Do not administer to clients with active liver disease, unexplained persistent elevations in serum transaminases, or to nursing or pregnant women.

- Monitor liver enzymes during therapy for possible hepatotoxicity.

- Assess for myopathy (muscle pain and weakness) and discontinue drug if this occurs.

- Advise client to immediately report unexplained skeletal muscle pain or weakness.

- Administer with caution concurrently with strong CYP3A4 enzyme inhibitors (such as clarithromycin, azole antifungals, grapefruit juice, or cyclosporine).

- Instruct women of childbearing age to use effective birth control method.

- Advise client to continue taking the drug, even if feeling fine.

- Advise client to limit or eliminate alcohol use during therapy because this increases the risk for hepatic toxicity.

- If concurrently taking warfarin, monitor INR regularly because simvastatin prolongs INR.

Generic: spironolactone (spir-OH-no-LAK-tone)

Brand: aldactone

Classification(s): Potassium-sparing diuretic; antihypertensive; aldosterone antagonist; electrolytic and water balance agent

Side Effects: Hyperkalemia, hyponatremia, gynecomastia, GI disturbances, drowsiness, headache, rash, confusion, drug fever, ataxia, impotence, hirsutism

Nursing Implications and Precautions:

- Do not administer to clients with hyperkalemia, renal impairment, or anuria.
- Administer with caution to clients with hepatic impairment, hyponatremia, or recent surgery.
- Monitor electrolytes; if hyperkalemia occurs, discontinue drug immediately.
- Advise client to avoid potassium supplements and potassium-containing salt substitutes.
- Concurrent administration of this drug with nonsteroidal anti-inflammatory drugs (NSAIDS) or ACE inhibitors can result in severe hyperkalemia.

- Advise client to limit or eliminate alcohol use during therapy because this increases side effects of the drug.
- Advise client to have blood pressure checked at regular intervals.
- Advise client to continue taking the drug, even if feeling fine.
- Advise client to avoid becoming overheated or dehydrated while exercising.

Generic: sulfamethoxazole+trimethoprim (sul-fah-meth-OX-ah-zole try-METH-oh-prim)

Brand: Bactrim, Septra

Classification(s): Urinary tract anti-infective; sulfonamide

Side Effects: GI upset, allergic skin reactions, blood dyscrasias, hemolysis, hepatic or renal toxicity, crystalluria, pancreatitis, photosensitivity, Stevens-Johnson syndrome, lupus-like syndrome

Nursing Implications and Precautions:

- Do not administer to clients with sulfonamide sensitivity, megaloblastic anemia due to folate deficiency, or during the third trimester of pregnancy (pregnancy Category C).

- Assess for history of hypersensitivity to sulfonamides or other antibiotics.

- Advise client to take drug for the entire length of time prescribed, even if symptoms of infection have resolved.

- Monitor for pseudomembranous colitis (severe diarrhea).

- Monitor blood, urine, and renal function during therapy.

- Administer with caution to clients with hepatic or renal impairment, AIDS, or folate or G6PD deficiency.

- Maintain adequate hydration to prevent crystalluria.

- Monitor for rash and discontinue drug if this occurs.

Generic: sumatriptan (soo-mah-TRIP-tan)

Brand: Imitrex

Classification(s): Antimigraine; serotonic 5-HT$_1$ receptor agonist

Side Effects: Tingling, flushing, dizziness, muscle pain/weakness, fatigue, drowsiness, anxiety, seizures, serious cardiac and cerebrovascular events (including fatalities), dysgeusia (with nasal spray)

Nursing Implications and Precautions:

- Do not administer to clients with myocardial infarction, angina pectoris, silent myocardial ischemia, stroke, TIA, ischemic bowel disease, vasospastic coronary artery disease, uncontrolled hypertension, or severe hepatic impairment.

- Do not administer concurrently with ergot-type drugs, other 5-HT$_1$ agonists or within 2 weeks after discontinuing MAO inhibitors.

- Monitor first dose, especially in clients with likelihood of unrecognized coronary artery disease.

- Monitor cardiovascular function with long-term use.

- Instruct client on proper use of autoinjector.

- Administer with caution to clients with hepatic or renal impairment or seizure risk.

- Advise client to avoid driving and other hazardous activities until the effects of the drug are known.

- Advise client that this drug should be used to treat a headache that has begun, and it is not effective in preventing headaches.

Generic: **tadalafil** (tay-DAL-ah-fill)

Brand: Cialis

Classification(s): Pulmonary antihypertensive; phosphodiesterase (PDE) inhibitor; vasodilator

Side Effects: Headache, flushing, dyspepsia, nasal congestion, visual disturbances, priapism

Nursing Implications and Precautions:

- Do not administer this drug to clients concurrently taking organic nitrates or sodium nitroprusside.
- Administer with caution to clients with myocardial infarction, stroke, or life-threatening arrhythmia within 6 months; blood pressure less than 90/50 mmHg or greater than 170/110 mmHg; unstable angina; left ventricular outflow obstruction; anatomical penile deformation; predisposition to priapism; bleeding disorders; active peptic ulcer; or retinitis pigmentosa.

- Monitor blood pressure during therapy in clients concurrently taking antihypertensives because the tadalafil may significantly lower blood pressure.
- Advise client to promptly seek medical attention if the drug causes a sudden loss of vision or hearing or if a painful erection lasts longer than 4 hours.
- Advise client not to share the medication.
- Advise client to take drug exactly as prescribed; the "as-needed" dose is higher than the "daily" dose.
- Advise client to take the drug 30–60 minutes prior to expected sexual activity.

Generic: **tamoxifen** (tam-OX-ih-fen)

Brand: Soltamox, Nolvadex

Classification(s): Antineoplastic; antiestrogen; selective estrogen receptor modifier (SERM)

Side Effects: Hot flashes, vaginal discharge, altered menses, rash, headache, nausea, cough, edema, fatigue, abdominal cramps, hypercalcemia, thrombotic events, ovarian cysts, uterine fibroids or cancer, visual changes, jaundice, hypertriglyceridemia, blood dyscrasias, hair loss

Nursing Implications and Precautions:

- Do not administer to clients with history of deep vein thrombosis or pulmonary embolism or to women who are nursing or pregnant (pregnancy Category D).

- Do not administer concurrently with coumarin-type anticoagulants because bleeding may occur.

- Advise client to have a gynecological exam at least annually.

- Monitor for increased risk of uterine cancer and thrombotic events.

- Advise client to immediately report symptoms of thromboembolic disease during therapy (chest pain, shortness of breath, pain in calves).

- Monitor serum calcium levels and discontinue if severe hypercalcemia occurs.

- Monitor blood, lipids, and liver function.

- Advise client to immediately report any new breast lumps or abnormal vaginal bleeding.

- If client is premenopausal, advise the use of nonhormonal contraception during and within 2 months of discontinuing therapy.

Generic: **tamsulosin** (tam-su-LOH-sin)

Brand: Flomax

Classification(s): Smooth muscle relaxant of bladder outlet and prostate gland; alpha-adrenergic receptor antagonist

Side Effects: Syncope (first-dose effect), headache, dizziness, drowsiness, rhinitis, blurred vision, orthostatic hypotension, asthenia, sexual disorders, insomnia, priapism (rare)

Nursing Implications and Precautions:

- Monitor blood pressure during therapy to evaluate drug effectiveness.

- Advise client to move slowly from a lying to a standing position to prevent light-headedness.

- Monitor client carefully for hypotension following the first dose and when dosages are increased.

- Advise client to take drug at bedtime to avoid drowsiness or dizziness.

- Advise the male client to immediately report a penis erection that is painful and lasts 4 hours or longer because this may result in permanent damage to erectile tissue.

- Administer with caution to clients with hepatic impairment.

- Assess for prostate cancer prior to treatment because this drug is contraindicated in these clients.

- Advise client to report changes in sexual performance, including abnormal ejaculation or decreased libido.

- Do not administer concurrently with strong CYP3A4 enzyme inhibitors (such as ketoconazole).

- Do not administer to clients who report a severe sensitivity to sulfa drugs.

Generic: temazepam (tem-AYZ-eh-pam)

Brand: Restoril

Classification(s): Antianxiety; sedative-hypnotic; benzodiazepine

Side Effects: Complex sleep-related behaviors, dizziness, ataxia, drowsiness, sedation, confusion, dependence, blurred vision, paradoxical excitement, fetal toxicity (pregnancy Category X)

Nursing Implications and Precautions:

- Do not administer to women who are pregnant or nursing.
- Advise the female client to immediately notify the prescriber of known or suspected pregnancy.
- Advise client to not discontinue the drug abruptly.
- Advise client to avoid driving and other hazardous activities until the effects of the drug are known.
- Administer with caution to clients with suicidal ideation, history of substance abuse, depression, and renal, hepatic, or respiratory impairment.
- Advise client to store drug in a safe place, away from children or those who may take the drug for recreational purposes.
- Advise client to limit or eliminate alcohol use during therapy because this will increase drowsiness.
- Use caution when administering other CNS depressants concurrently due to the potential for excessive sedation.
- Assess for signs of overdose or abuse (confusion, sedation, slurred speech, coma).
- Evaluate drug effectiveness for treating insomnia after 7–10 days; failure to resolve symptoms may indicate the presence of a primary psychiatric disorder or other illness that needs evaluation.
- Advise client to take the drug immediately prior to expected sleep.

Generic: terazosin (terr-AY-zoh-sin)

Brand: Hytrin

Classification(s): Antihypertensive benign prostatic hypertrophy agent; alpha-adrenergic receptor antagonist

Side Effects: Syncope (first-dose effect), dizziness, drowsiness, fatigue, dyspnea, rhinitis, blurred vision, orthostatic hypotension, asthenia, priapism (rare)

Nursing Implications and Precautions:

- Monitor blood pressure during therapy to evaluate drug effectiveness.

- Advise client to move slowly from a lying to a standing position to prevent light-headedness.

- Monitor client carefully for hypotension following the first dose and when dosages are increased.

- Advise client to take drug at bedtime to avoid drowsiness or dizziness.

- Advise the male client to immediately report a penis erection that is painful and lasts 4 hours or longer because this may result in permanent damage to erectile tissue.

- Administer with caution to clients with hepatic impairment.

- Assess for prostate cancer prior to treatment because this drug is contraindicated in these clients.

- Administer with caution to clients concurrently taking verapamil or other antihypertensives.

Generic: testosterone (tess-TOS-ter-own)

Brand: Striant, Testoderm, Teslac, Androgel, Androderm

Classification(s): Antineoplastic; androgen/anabolic steroid

Generic: tiotropium (tye-oh-TROH-pee-um)

Brand: Spiriva

Classification(s): Bronchodilator; antispasmodic; anticholinergic; antimuscarinic

Side Effects: Local reactions (topical applications), headache, increased hemoglobin/hematocrit or blood pressure, depression, hot flashes, insomnia, mood swings, virilization

Nursing Implications and Precautions:

- Do not administer to men with breast or prostate cancer.
- Advise pregnant and nursing women to avoid contact of the drug with skin (pregnancy Category X).
- Monitor for prostate enlargement or cancer during therapy, especially in older adult men.
- Administer with caution to clients with cardiac, renal, or hepatic disease or sleep apnea.

- Monitor hemoglobin, hematocrit, and serum lipids during therapy.
- Advise client to avoid showering or swimming for at least 2 hours after application of topical forms.
- Monitor liver function during therapy and discontinue drug if impairment occurs.

Side Effects: Paradoxical bronchospasm, dyspepsia, headache, dry mouth, upper respiratory tract infection, allergy, rhinitis

Nursing Implications and Precautions:

- Teach client proper use of the inhaler device.
- Advise client that this drug should not be used to treat an acute asthma attack that has already begun.
- Administer with caution to clients with narrow-angle glaucoma or urinary retention.
- Advise client to take drug exactly as prescribed and not use larger doses without consulting with the prescriber.

- Advise client to keep track of the number of sprays used and to obtain refills before 200 sprays are reached.
- Advise client to continue taking the drug, even if feeling better.
- Advise client that the drug is for inhalation only and to not swallow the capsules.

Generic: tizanidine (tye-ZAN-ih-deen)

Brand: Zanaflex

Classification(s): Central-acting skeletal muscle relaxant; antispasmodic

Generic: tolterodine (tol-TER-oh-deen)

Brand: Detrol

Classification(s): Antimuscarinic; bladder antispasmodic; anticholinergic

Side Effects: Dry mouth, somnolence, asthenia, dizziness, urinary tract infection, elevated liver enzymes, vomiting, blurred vision, dyskinesia, nervousness, hypotension

Nursing Implications and Precautions:

- Do not administer concurrently with concomitant fluvoxamine or ciprofloxacin.
- Administer with caution to clients with hepatic or renal impairment and cardiovascular disease.
- Monitor ophthalmic and liver function regularly.
- Advise client to move slowly from a lying to a standing position to prevent light-headedness.
- Advise client to not discontinue the drug abruptly.
- Monitor blood pressure during therapy, especially in clients concurrently taking antihypertensives.
- Advise client to limit or eliminate alcohol use during therapy because this may cause excessive drowsiness.
- Advise client to avoid driving and other hazardous activities until the effects of the drug are known.

Side Effects: Dyspepsia, anticholinergic effects (dry mouth, dizziness, blurred vision, constipation, nausea), fatigue

Nursing Implications and Precautions:

- Do not administer to clients with uncontrolled narrow-angle glaucoma or urinary or gastric retention.
- Administer with caution to clients with myasthenia gravis, Q-T prolongation, bladder outflow obstruction, or gastrointestinal obstruction.
- Advise client to avoid driving and other hazardous activities until the effects of the drug are known.
- Advise client to limit or eliminate alcohol use during therapy because this may cause excessive drowsiness.
- Advise client to notify health care providers of all medications taken because tolterodine interacts with multiple drugs.
- Advise clients taking extended-release forms to swallow the drug whole and not to crush, split, or chew the capsules.

Generic: topiramate (toe-PEER-ah-mate)

Brand: Topamax

Classification(s): Anticonvulsant; antiepileptic; gamma-aminobutyrate (GABA) enhancer

Side Effects: Drowsiness, dizziness, ataxia, speech disorder, psychomotor slowing, nervousness, other mental changes, paresthesia, fatigue, weight loss, GI upset, anorexia

Nursing Implications and Precautions:

- Administer with caution to clients with renal or hepatic impairment or kidney stones.
- Monitor for acute myopia and angle closure glaucoma because untreated elevated intraocular pressure can lead to permanent visual loss.
- Monitor for decreased sweating and increased body temperature, especially in pediatric clients.
- Monitor for suicidal ideation.
- Monitor serum bicarbonate to prevent metabolic acidosis.
- Monitor for depression and other behavioral changes during therapy.

- Advise client to avoid driving and other hazardous activities until the effects of the drug are known.
- Advise client to not discontinue the drug abruptly because this may cause seizures.
- Advise client to limit or eliminate alcohol use during therapy because this may cause excessive drowsiness.
- Advise client to immediately report any eye pain or sudden changes in vision.

Generic: tramadol (TRAM-ah-doll)

Brand: Ultram

Classification(s): Narcotic analgesic

Side Effects: Dizziness, GI upset, constipation, headache, somnolence, pruritus, CNS stimulation, asthenia, sweating, dry mouth, seizures, anaphylaxis

Nursing Implications and Precautions:

- Do not administer to clients with acute intoxication with alcohol, hypnotics, centrally-acting analgesics, opioids, or psychotropic drugs.

- Administer with caution to clients with respiratory depression, increased intracranial pressure, head injury, seizure disorders, acute abdomen, renal or hepatic impairment, or suicidal ideation.

- Monitor carefully in clients with high potential for substance abuse.

- Monitor for interactions with other CNS depressants.

- Monitor for excessive sedation.

- Advise client to avoid driving and other hazardous activities until the effects of the drug are known.

- Advise client to limit or eliminate alcohol use during therapy because this may cause excessive drowsiness.

- Monitor for increased seizure activity.

- Advise client to not discontinue the drug abruptly because this will cause withdrawal symptoms.

- Advise client to store drug in a safe place, away from children or those who may take the drug for recreational purposes.

Generic: trazodone (TRAZ-oh-doan)

Brand: Desyrel

Classification(s): Antidepressant

Side Effects: Suicidal ideation, drowsiness, dizziness, constipation, blurred vision, orthostatic hypotension, abnormal bleeding, priapism, serotonin syndrome (rare), neuroleptic malignant syndrome (rare)

Nursing Implications and Precautions:

* Do not administer to clients with suicidal ideation.

* Monitor for worsening depression, unusual behavioral changes, and suicidal ideation.

* Advise client to continue taking the drug, even if feeling better.

* Do not administer this drug to clients taking monoamine oxidase (MAO) inhibitors.

* Advise client to not discontinue the drug abruptly.

* Monitor for occult gastrointestinal (GI) bleeding.

* Advise client to not take aspirin or other drugs that affect coagulation, unless directed by the prescriber.

* Advise client to limit or eliminate alcohol use during therapy because this increases drowsiness.

* Administer with caution to clients with heart disease because this drug may increase the risk for arrhythmias.

* Advise the male client to immediately report a penis erection that is painful and lasts 4 hours or longer because this may result in permanent damage to erectile tissue.

Generic: triamcinolone inhaler (try-am-SIN-oh-lone)

Brand: Nasacort AQ, Azmacort

Classification(s): Anti-inflammatory; immunosuppressant; adrenal corticosteroid; glucocorticoid

Generic: triamcinolone topical (try-am-SIN-oh-lone)

Brand: Kenalog

Classification(s): Anti-inflammatory; immunosuppressant; adrenal corticosteroid; glucocorticoid

Side Effects: Headache, pharyngitis, epistaxis, nasal burning, asthma symptoms, GI upset, cough

Nursing Implications and Precautions:

- Advise client to take drug for the entire length of time prescribed, even if symptoms have resolved.
- Monitor for adrenal insufficiency if client is concurrently receiving other systemic or topical corticosteroids.
- Advise client to take drug exactly as prescribed and not to take it more frequently.
- Monitor for localized *Candida* infection and other nasal mucosal changes.
- Administer with caution to clients with tuberculosis or other infections such as chickenpox, measles, or ocular herpes simplex.
- If exposed to measles or chickenpox, consider anti-infective prophylactic therapy. Monitor for growth reduction in children.
- Advise client that Azmacort is not intended for treatment of acute asthma attack.

Side Effects: Local burning, stinging, pruritus, erythema, skin atrophy, striae, miliaria, secondary infections, hypopigmentation, folliculitis, acneiform eruptions, contact dermatitis

Nursing Implications and Precautions:

- Do not use this drug to treat viral infections.
- Avoid contact with eyes, diaper dermatitis, or pre-existing skin atrophy.
- Do not apply to large areas of denuded, broken, or inflamed skin.
- Avoid using occlusive dressings after applying the drug.
- For prolonged or extensive therapy, monitor for Cushing's syndrome; substitute a lower potency form of the drug if this occurs.

Generic: triamterene+hydrochlorothiazide (HCTZ)
(try-AM-tare-een hy-dro-klor-oh-THI-ah-zide)

Brand: Dyazide, Maxzide

Classification(s): Potassium-sparing diuretic; electrolyte and water balance agent

Generic: valacyclovir (val-ah-SYE-klo-veer)

Brand: Valtrex

Classification(s): Antiviral

Side Effects: Drowsiness, muscle cramps, weakness, headache, GI disturbances, dizziness, arrhythmias, hypotension, dry mouth, urine discoloration

Nursing Implications and Precautions:

- Do not administer to clients with renal impairment, hyperkalemia, or sulfonamide allergy.
- Administer with caution to clients with hepatic dysfunction, diabetes, gout, asthma, history of kidney stones, or metabolic acidosis.
- Monitor electrolytes; if hyperkalemia occurs, discontinue drug immediately.
- Advise client to not use potassium supplements and potassium-containing salt substitutes.

- Monitor periodic blood glucose levels in clients with diabetes.
- Advise client to limit or eliminate alcohol use during therapy because this increases the risk of orthostatic hypotension.
- Advise client to avoid becoming overheated or dehydrated while exercising.
- Advise client to have blood pressure checked at regular intervals.

Side Effects: Headache, nausea, fatigue, allergic reaction, dizziness

Nursing Implications and Precautions:

- Advise client to take drug for the entire length of time prescribed, even if lesions are healing or disappear.
- Monitor for thrombotic thrombocytopenic purpura/ hemolytic uremic syndrome (TTP/HUS).
- Monitor for acute renal failure.

- Monitor for central nervous system adverse reactions (e.g., agitation, hallucinations, confusion, and encephalopathy), especially in older adult clients.
- Advise client to begin therapy as soon as possible after symptoms appear.

Generic: valsartan (val-SAR-tan)

Brand: Diovan

Classification(s): Antihypertensive; angiotensin receptor antagonist

Generic: vancomycin (van-ko-MYE-sin)

Brand: Vancocin

Classification(s): Antibiotic; glycopeptide

Side Effects: Viral infection, dizziness, abdominal pain, fatigue, hypotension, rhabdomyolysis (rare), fetal death and injury

Nursing Implications and Precautions:

- Instruct women of childbearing age to use effective birth control method (pregnancy Category D in second and third trimesters).

- Advise the female client to immediately notify the prescriber of known or suspected pregnancy.

- Monitor blood pressure during therapy to evaluate drug effectiveness.

- Advise client to take drug for the entire length of time prescribed, even if feeling better.

- Assess electrolytes and correct salt or volume depletion prior to starting therapy.

- Administer with caution to clients with renal or hepatic impairment, heart failure, or renal artery stenosis.

- Advise client not to use salt substitutes containing potassium, unless directed by the prescriber.

- Monitor for myopathy and discontinue drug if symptoms of muscle pain or weakness persist.

Side Effects: Nausea, drug fever, urticaria, rash (may be Stevens-Johnson syndrome), ototoxicity, nephrotoxicity, neutropenia, anaphylaxis, interstitial nephritis, vertigo

Nursing Implications and Precautions:

- Administer with caution to clients with renal insufficiency, colitis, or inflammatory bowel disorders.

- Monitor hearing during therapy.

- Monitor complete blood counts during therapy.

- Monitor renal function during therapy.

- Administer with caution when used concomitantly with other nephrotoxic or ototoxic drugs.

- Monitor injection site for possible extravasation, which can be very painful and damaging to the tissue.

- Administer drug over a period of at least 60 minutes to avoid rapid infusion-related reactions.

- Monitor for pseudomembranous colitis (severe diarrhea).

Generic: varenicline (ver-EN-ih-kleen)

Brand: Chantix

Classification(s): Smoking deterrent; nicotinic receptor agonist

Side Effects: Nausea; vivid, unusual, or strange dreams; constipation, flatulence, and vomiting; serious neuropsychiatric symptoms, including behavioral changes, agitation, depression, and suicidal ideation

Nursing Implications and Precautions:

- Monitor for edema and other serious allergic reactions.
- Monitor for serious skin rashes.
- Advise client to avoid driving and other hazardous activities until the effects of the drug are known.
- Administer with caution to clients with psychiatric disorders and renal impairment.
- Monitor for behavioral changes and suicidal ideation and discontinue drug immediately if these occur.
- Advise client that the normal time of therapy is 12 weeks, although longer therapy is sometimes warranted.

Generic: venlafaxine (VEN-lah-fax-een)

Brand: Effexor

Classification(s): Antidepressant; serotonin norepinephrine reuptake inhibitor (SNRI)

Side Effects: Abnormalities in sexual function, nausea, dry mouth, drowsiness, dizziness, sweating, constipation, nervousness, tremor, anorexia, blurred vision, suicidal ideation, hypertension, serotonin syndrome (rare) and neuroleptic malignant syndrome (rare)

Nursing Implications and Precautions:

- Do not administer to clients with suicidal ideation.
- Monitor for worsening depression, unusual behavioral changes, and suicidal ideation.
- Advise client to continue taking the drug, even if feeling better.
- Do not administer this drug to clients taking monoamine oxidase (MAO) inhibitors.
- Advise client to not discontinue the drug abruptly.

- Advise client to not take aspirin or other drugs that affect coagulation unless directed by the prescriber.
- Advise client to limit or eliminate alcohol use during therapy because this increases drowsiness.
- Advise the client to report changes in sexual function, including delayed ejaculation, impotence, and loss of libido.
- Advise client that the drug must be taken at least 4 weeks before its full effects are noticed.

Generic: verapamil (verr-AP-ah-mill)

Brand: Calan, others

Classification(s): Antiarrhythmic (class IV); antihypertensive; antianginal; calcium channel blocker

Side Effects: Constipation, hypotension, headache, dizziness, peripheral edema, nausea

Nursing Implications and Precautions:

* Assess for swelling of hands, feet, and ankles.

* Administer with caution to clients with bradycardia, sick sinus syndrome, heart failure, or hepatic impairment.

* Monitor blood pressure periodically to ensure drug effectiveness.

* Advise client to continue taking the drug, even if symptoms resolve.

* Advise client to limit or eliminate alcohol use during therapy.

* Advise client to move slowly from a lying to a standing position to prevent light-headedness.

* Monitor client carefully when beginning therapy or changing doses because this may worsen angina pain or cause a myocardial infarction.

* Advise clients taking extended-release forms to swallow the drug whole and not to crush, split, or chew the capsules.

Generic: warfarin (WAR-fah-rin)

Brand: Coumadin

Classification(s): Anticoagulant

Side Effects: Tissue or organ hemorrhage, skin or tissue necrosis, allergic reactions, systemic cholesterol microembolization, purple toes syndrome, vasculitis, hepatic disorders, fever, dermatitis, urticaria, abdominal pain

Nursing Implications and Precautions:

- Do not administer warfarin to clients with hemorrhagic conditions or treatments, malignant hypertension, blood dyscrasias, recent surgery, major regional, lumbar block anesthesia, or spinal puncture.
- Monitor PT/INR regularly.
- Administer with caution to clients with hepatic or renal insufficiency, infection, trauma, diabetes, hypertension, heart failure, edema, hyperlipidemia, thyroid disorders, collagen vascular disease, protein C deficiency, heparin-induced thrombocytopenia, polycythemia vera, cancer, vasculitis, indwelling catheter, fever, gangrene, diarrhea, or dental procedures.

- Advise client that risk for bleeding may continue for 2–5 days after discontinuation of the drug.
- Monitor for tissue necrosis or systemic cholesterol microembolization and discontinue drug if these occur.
- Advise client to immediately report any signs of unusual bruising or bleeding.
- Advise client to notify health care providers of all medications taken because warfarin interacts with multiple drugs.

Generic: **zidovudine** (zye-DOE-vyoo-deen)

Brand: AZT, Retrovir

Classification(s): Antiviral; nucleoside reverse transcriptase inhibitor

Side Effects: Anemia, neutropenia, headache, malaise, GI disturbances, myopathy, neuropathy, myositis, thrombocytopenia, lactic acidosis, steatosis, hepatomegaly, fat redistribution, immune reconstitution syndrome, pancreatitis

Nursing Implications and Precautions:

- Monitor liver function and discontinue drug if lactic acidosis, hepatomegaly, or steatosis occurs.

- Advise client to immediately report symptoms of liver disease (nausea/vomiting, diarrhea, anorexia, stomach pain, low fever, dark urine, clay-colored stools, or jaundice).

- Monitor blood counts for hematologic toxicity and discontinue drug if significant anemia or granulocytopenia occurs.

- Advise client to notify health care providers of all medications taken because zidovudine interacts with multiple drugs.

- Administer with caution to clients with bone marrow suppression.

Generic: zolpidem (zole-PIH-dem)

Brand: Ambien

Classification(s): Sedative-hypnotic; antianxiety; non-benzodiazepine

Side Effects: Dizziness, headache, nervousness, complex sleep-related behaviors

Nursing Implications and Precautions:

- Administer with caution to clients with depression, behavioral changes, compromised respiratory function, or conditions that affect metabolism or hemodynamic response.

- Monitor carefully in clients with high potential for substance abuse.

- Advise client to not discontinue the drug abruptly.

- Advise client not to drive or operate hazardous machinery until the effects of the drug are known.

- Advise client that the drug must be taken several weeks before the full effects of the drug are noticed.

- Advise client to limit or eliminate alcohol use during therapy because this increases drowsiness.

- Evaluate drug effectiveness for treating insomnia after 7–10 days; failure to resolve symptoms may indicate the presence of a primary psychiatric disorder or other illness that needs evaluation.

- Advise client to take the drug immediately prior to expected sleep.

Appendix

Common Sound-Alike/ Look-Alike Medications

Aciphex/Aricept
Actonel/Actos
Advair/Advicor
Alprazolam/Lorazepam
Amiloride/Amlodipine
Aminophylline/Amiodarone
Avinza/Evista
Benazapril/Benadryl
Bupropion/Buspirone
Carbamazepine/Oxcarbazepine
Celebrex/Celexa
Clomiphene/Clomipramine
Cozaar/Zocor
Dilaudid/Dilantin
Diprivan/Diflucan
Doxorubicin/Daunorubicin
Felodipine/Famotidine
Fluoxetine/Duloxetine
Glyburide/Glipizide
HCTZ/HCTZ-triamterene
Hydralazine/Hydroxyzine
Imuran/Imdur
Klonopin/Clonidine
Lamictal/Lamisil
Lamivudine/Lamotrigene
Ludiomil/Lomotil
Levothyroxine/Levaquin
Loratadine/Lorazepam
Macrobid/Macrodantin
Maxzide/Microzide
Methohexital/Methotrexate

Metocurine/Metoclopramide
Midodrine/Midrin
Mirapex/Miralax
Mucomyst/Mucinex
Neulasta/Neumega
Nicardipine/Nifedipine
Oxybutynin/Oxycodone
Oxycodone/Hydrocodone
Paxil/Doxil
Penicillamine/Penicillin
Prednisone/Prednisolone
Procanbid/Probenecid
Procarbazine/Procardia
Propofol/Propranolol
Quinidine/Quinine
Restoril/Risperdal
Rifaximin/Rifampin
Serophene/Sarafem
Seroquel/Serzone
Simvastatin/Simethicone
Sufentanil/Fentanyl
Sulfasalazine/Salsalate
Sulfasalazine/Sulfadiazine
Sumatriptan/Zolmitriptan
Tacrolimus/Tacrine
Taxol/Paxil
Topamax/Toprol-XL
Torsemide/Toradol
Vinblastine/Vincristine
Vioxx/Zyvox
Zolpidem/Zolmitriptan

Index

Notes

Installing the Anki Software for REA's NCLEX-RN Flashcards

System Requirements: Windows XP or later, MacOSX (all versions)

Installers for the operating systems above are included on the CD. Installers for numerous other devices and operating systems, including Linux, Android, and iPhone are available for download at *http://www.ankisrs.net.*

To install the Anki Learning System, insert the CD in your computer's CD or DVD drive.

Windows Users:
- Double-click on My Computer, and double-click on your CD-ROM drive
- Double-click on the file named Anki-1.0.1.exe, and follow the on-screen instructions
- Follow the instructions below to import REA's NCLEX-RN Vocabulary and Medications Flashcards
- Click File, then choose Save to save the deck after importation

Mac OS Users:
- Double-click on the CD-ROM icon on your desktop
- Double-click on the file named Anki-1.0.1.dmg, then double-click on the Anki disk image on your desktop
- Copy the Anki application and REA's-NCLEX-RN-Vocabulary-and-Medications.anki to your applications folder
- Launch the application from your Applications folder, then follow the import instructions below

Importing REA's *NCLEX-RN Vocabulary & Medications Flashcards*
- Launch the Anki Learning System
- From the File Menu, click Import
- Browse to your CD or DVD drive
- Using the pull-down menu, change the file type to Anki Deck (*.anki)
- Choose REA's *NCLEX-RN Vocabulary and Medications Flashcards* from the list
- Anki will then import your flashcards.

To begin studying, click the Start Reviewing button.

The Anki Learning System allows you to rate your confidence level for each card. Cards that you rate with a low confidence rating (Again) will be shown again soon, while cards with a high confidence rating will be shown less frequently (Easy).

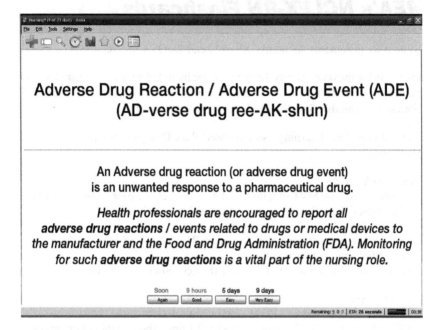

Technical Support

For more information about adding cards, editing cards, or resetting your data, click the Help menu, and choose Documentation.

For full documentation and a list of frequently asked questions, visit *http://www.ankisrs.net.*

If you have questions regarding the content of REA's *NCLEX-RN Vocabulary and Medications Flashcards*, please contact REA at *info@rea.com.*

Note: REA's Anatomy charts are included on the CD in a folder named Reference Charts.